Progression**Series**

Medicine
and Dentistry

For entry to university and college in 2007

PUBLISHED BY: UCAS ROSEHILL NEW BARN LANE CHELTENHAM GL52 3LZ

PRODUCED IN CONJUNCTION WITH GTI SPECIALIST PUBLISHERS

ISBN: 1-84361-058-2

UCAS REFERENCE NUMBER: DI102/07
PUBLICATION REFERENCE: 06_056

FURTHER COPIES AVAILABLE FROM WWW.UCASBOOKS.COM

POST: UCAS MEDIA PO BOX 130 CHELTENHAM GL52 3ZF
T: +44 (0)1242 544610   F: +44 (0)1242 544806

FURTHER INFORMATION ABOUT THE UCAS APPLICATION PROCESS
T: +44 (0)870 1122211   F: +44 (0)1242 544961

PRINTED BY THE CROMWELL PRESS, TROWBRIDGE, WILTSHIRE.

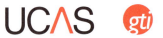

Foreword

THINKING ABOUT MEDICINE AND DENTISTRY

Researching the type of course you would like to study at higher education level means that you are half way towards choosing the right qualification for you. Knowing which subject or subjects you would enjoy is a distinct advantage, but each course can vary depending on the specific areas covered and the university or college you choose to attend. Even if the course title is the same at a number of institutions, it does not mean that the content or teaching methods will be the same. Finding a university or college that will suit you academically and personally can take time. Throughout the year, there are opportunities to visit the different universities and colleges, where advisers can tell you about the courses in detail and you can see where you will be living and studying for the next few years of your life.

Speaking to former students of the course you would like to study is extremely useful – they can give you an insider's view of university life and the teaching standards that you could not find anywhere else. We at UCAS have teamed up with GTI Specialist Publishers to provide the careers advice and real-life case studies in this publication. You will find information on becoming a doctor or dentist, how to study medicine and dentistry and medicine and dentistry course listings. We hope you find this publication helps you to choose a course and university that are right for you.

On behalf of UCAS and GTI Specialist Publishers, I wish you every success in your research.

Anthony McClaran, Chief Executive, UCAS

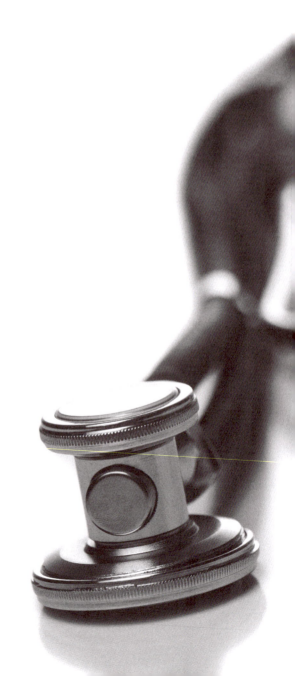

ProgressionSeries

Why medicine or dentistry?

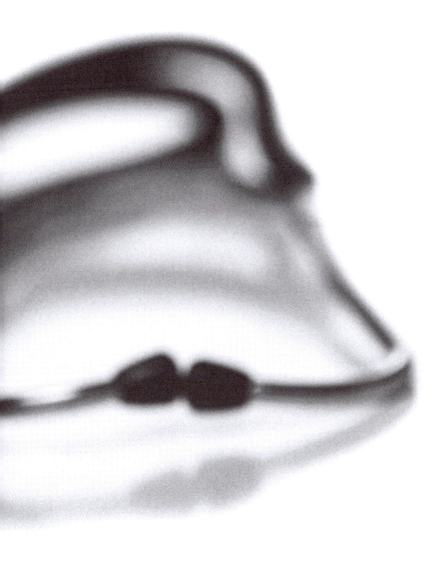

It could be you…

Reviving a stroke victim, then a partygoer who's had a bit too much to drink	— A&E
Using image diagnostics to spot the source of internal bleeding	— Radiology
Going in and stopping the internal bleeding at its source	— Surgery
Performing an emergency Caesarean section to save a baby's life	— Obstetrics
Listening to a new mum struggling with post-natal depression	— Psychiatry
Six colds, three pregnant mums and two cancer sufferers all in one afternoon	— GP
Ten fillings, three extractions, two bridges, five crowns	— Dentist

…and lots more besides. From your first filling to your first child to your first bereavement, doctors and dentists will feature in your life as helpers, even life-savers, and support. Some you will meet only briefly for those one-off emergency or consultation encounters. Others, like your GP and family dentist, will be with you for longer. Could a career as a dentist or doctor be for you? The aim of this guide is to help you decide.

A CAREER IN MEDICINE OR DENTISTRY?

- A qualified GP can earn £70,000+ – see 'A Career in Medicine' on page 16
- Over 70% of dentists are general dental practitioners – see 'A Career in Dentistry' on page 26
- As well as your academic ability, admissions tutors look for people skills, decisiveness, calmness under fire, attention to detail – see 'The Career For You?' on page 37
- Qualifying as a doctor takes 9-15 years full-time – see 'Routes to Qualification' on page 48

MEDICINE

It's an exciting time to train as a doctor in the UK. As part of the Department of Health's Modernising Medical Careers initiative, a two-year foundation programme will replace the existing pre-registration house officer (PRHO) year and the first senior house officer (SHO) year. Every postgraduate trainee will have a structured programme of managed education that should allow them to experience training placements in clinical areas that have not previously been accessible. On satisfactory completion of the foundation programme, doctors can enter specialist training, which will equip them with the qualifications to become either a consultant or a GP. For more information and updates, see www.mmc.nhs.uk.

DENTISTRY

People decide on dentistry for very different reasons:

- for some, it's the appeal of the 'fiddly' or the creative and aesthetic side of dentistry
- for others, it's a more sociable option than medicine, since you get to form long-term relationships with your patients and provide them with continuing care
- for others, the decision's made for practical reasons – qualifying as a general practice dentist costs less and doesn't take as long as the medical route.

Whatever the reason, dentistry offers **an increasingly broad range of career options, a stable future** – since dentists are so in demand in the UK, and a very **flexible type of employment** (dentists can set their own working hours).

If you're interested in a possible career in medicine or dentistry, then this guide can help point you further in the right direction. Read on to discover:

- the main areas of work and roles on offer
- what it takes to be a doctor or a dentist
- how to get in and the paths to qualification
- advice from trainee and practising doctors and dentists.

Why medicine or dentistry?

Choose a career that is...

VARIED

There are few careers that offer as much variety as medicine and dentistry – both in the potential areas of work and your day-to-day experiences. Once you've chosen your specialism – and that includes being a GP or family dentist – new drugs and technology mean your career is constantly refreshed as you face new challenges and learn new techniques. And even if the medical problems are the same, the people affected by them will be **very** different.

VITAL TO SOCIETY

There are around 12 million admissions to hospital in England each year, with over a third of these being emergencies. Medicine and dentistry are so important to society that the government spent around £75 billion on the NHS in 2005/6, making it the second-largest government spending programme. But their importance isn't just a matter of statistics. How recently did someone in your family see a doctor or dentist? Or when did you last hear about someone making a miraculous recovery from illness, or benefiting from life-changing surgery, or even having a troublesome tooth removed? As a doctor or a dentist, you'll really make a difference.

TECHNICAL AND PEOPLE-FOCUSED

Many careers appeal because of the chance to develop technical expertise or to work with people. In medicine or dentistry you can lean towards one of these, but you will need a balance and interest in both. You'll use the latest drugs and technology, but you'll also see how these affect real people – **your** patients.

(LARGELY) WELL PAID

It can be a long and expensive process to reach fully qualified status, but the financial rewards are there. Both doctors and dentists receive above-average earnings throughout their careers. As a trainee doctor or dentist, your annual salary could be over £30,000, and at consultant level it could reach £90,000. Check out the salary levels on pages 18 (medicine) and 27 (dentistry) for more information.

SECURE IN THE LONG-TERM

People will always get ill, break their legs playing football or have something go wrong with their teeth, so your skills, knowledge and expertise will always be in demand. Both medicine and dentistry also have clearly structured career paths and you won't necessarily be tied to one hospital, practice or location either. There are around 180 NHS acute trusts (providing medical and surgical care) and 250 private sector hospitals in the UK, many of which are national centres of excellence for different specialisms, so you don't **have** to work in London.

WHAT DO TRAINEE MEDICS AND DENTISTS SAY?

"I love coming to work and seeing patients. Wonderful!"

Uma Kannan, 34, GP registrar

"I feel confident that I have the professional and social skills to treat any patient who might walk through the door."

Nicole Marriott, 23, vocational dental practitioner

"I wanted to do a job in which I could serve people and share their problems."

Syed Arsalan Raza, 27, trainee doctor (foundation year two)

"I've always looked for a challenge. And around the time I was making decisions about my career, I was really starting to enjoy biology, so medicine was an obvious choice."

Mark Hohenberg, 24, sixth-year medical student

"I worked as a dental nurse to fund my gap year. After a few months I could see how much job satisfaction dentistry offered and decided to train to become a dentist."

Rupert Austin, 24, fifth-year dental student

"I don't like being bored, so I wanted to work in an area that would challenge me and where I could learn on the job. I wanted to do something scientific and be able to make a difference."

Ed Hyde, 24, trainee doctor (foundation year two)

Medicine or dentistry?

Find out more about each profession before you make your choice.

MEDICINE

Doctors take the science of medicine, ie how our bodies and minds work, and use it to help people deal with disease, pain and ill health.

What types of doctors are there?

There are over 60 medical specialities available to doctors once they have completed their general medical training. They have many requirements and characteristics in common, but some require particular skills, eg manual dexterity for surgery, and each requires doctors to take specialist exams. Each specialty is governed by a Royal College or Faculty, which sets the entry and training requirements and the specialist membership and fellowship exams. (See 'Which specialism?' on page 21).

Where could you work?

There are over 100,000 doctors in the UK, the vast majority of whom are employed in the NHS. However, many (particularly fully qualified consultants) now also work either exclusively in private sector hospitals or across both the public and private sectors. NHS doctors will either work in a hospital (for example, as an orthopaedic surgeon) or in a community setting (for example a general practitioner). An alternative route is to be sponsored by the armed forces – for example, as an RAF or Royal Navy medical officer. Your fees and salary will be paid throughout your training in exchange for a commitment to a minimum period of service, after which you can decide to stay or leave.

DENTISTRY

Dentists are healthcare professionals who are experts in the diagnosis and treatment of a range of problems affecting the mouth and teeth. The most effective dentists combine strong **diagnostic**, **clinical** and **social** skills.

Where do they work?

General dental practice: Armed with a BDS (degree in dentistry) and just one year's practical postgraduate training in an approved practice (known as vocational training or VT), you could become a general dental practitioner, for example, in a local family or community practice. It's usual to work as an associate in someone else's practice before being able to set up on your own. Later on you could become a practice owner (principal) by becoming a partner, buying a practice or establishing a new practice. Once you've completed your training, you're pretty much up and running, and there are no higher grades or levels. This can be perceived as a relative lack of career progression, but the upside is that you can further your knowledge at your own pace and follow the particular dental specialities that interest you. And dentists start to earn good money much sooner than their medical colleagues. (However, their medical colleagues can overtake them on their way to a consultant position.)

As a general dental practitioner (GDP) you may practise under the NHS or privately. Many dentists opt for a mixture of NHS and private work. In private practice you may be more likely to perform a higher proportion of cosmetic dentistry alongside the more routine work. Under a new system introduced in England and Wales in April 2006, payment for NHS work is based on the amount of treatment carried out by each practice or practitioner. Private fees are set by each dentist individually and may vary according to the particular practice. As a GDP you are self-employed and running a business.

The armed forces: The Defence Dental Services sponsor a number of dental trainees through their undergraduate and vocational training and pay a salary to dental trainees in exchange for a commitment to work in the forces as a dentist for a certain period of time (for example, six years). Dentists in the armed forces hold a commissioned rank and have a very structured career path. The salary structure during the vocational period is different from that for the other options outlined on this page. For more information visit the Defence Dental Services website at www.dmsd.mod.uk/dda.htm.

Hospital dentistry: There are many specialisms if you go down this route, including orthodontics (bone structure), periodontics (gums) and surgical dentistry. Dental departments of large general hospitals have the facilities to offer treatment that may not be available or feasible in your local practice. You will tend to see fewer patients than in general practice, but their treatment is likely to be more complex. Unlike would-be GDPs you won't have to do the year of vocational training, but you will have to take the medical training route instead. There is a defined salary structure, career structure and training pathway for hospital dentists and you will need to obtain recognised postgraduate qualifications in order to advance.

Community dental service (CDS): Dentists working for a CDS provide care for patients with special needs – for example, elderly housebound people or those with mental or physical disabilities. To become a community dental officer, a graduate must also complete a period of vocational training. As in hospital dentistry, posts are salaried. There is a defined career structure and opportunities for managerial and research duties.

DENTISTS AT A GLANCE

- Mostly in general practice – over 70%
- Mostly men – approximately 67%

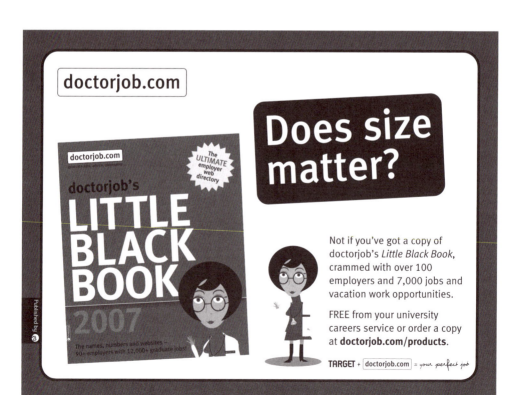

Introducing medicine

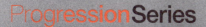

A career in medicine

This section aims to give you an overview of the main career choices, specialisms, working conditions and pay for doctors in the UK today.

If you have an interest in science and a desire to help people, then a career in medicine could be for you. At this stage in your career you don't need to decide on a particular specialty – most medical students choose once they've had had more exposure to the different fields of medicine during their medical course.

HOSPITAL DOCTOR OR GENERAL PRACTITIONER (GP)?

The most obvious choice for trainee doctors is between hospital and GP practice. GPs have less intensity of pressure, a chance to take more of a holistic approach to the treatment of their patients and more pay early on. Hospital doctors are at the leading edge, making an immediate impact on their patients' lives. The following chart sums up some of the key differences between the two roles.

HOSPITAL DOCTOR

- Mostly employed in NHS hospitals serving vast regional or even national populations; many also now work across public and private sectors
- More likely to be **specialist**
- One-off patient contact; sees patients for short intense periods
- **Hospital-based**
- Aspires to 'consultant', ie top expert in their specialism

GP

- Mostly employed by NHS local communities, serving a much smaller base of local people
- **Generalist**
  Ongoing patient contact; gets to know patients over time
- **Surgery-based**
  Aspires to 'GP Principal', ie senior partner in their practice

Working conditions

Flexible options such as job share, shared on-call, and part-time working are now available to trainee doctors once they've completed their university course.
This makes a medical career much more appealing to people who previously might have opted out of medicine due to the long working hours. This said, part-time is more readily available in some specialities than others. Working hours for junior doctors will be reduced to 56 hours per week in 2007, thanks to the EU Working Time Directive, and are due to be reduced further still. However, the work is still highly pressurised in some specialisms due to patient targets and altered working patterns.

Pay

As one medical registrar puts it, 'The money comes, but not quickly.' For hospital doctors, pay builds from a small beginning, offering great rewards to doctors as they near the top of their profession. GPs typically earn more money more quickly. There was some controversy surrounding the below-inflation pay rises awarded to doctors in 2005. At the time of preparing this guide, pay scales for 2006 had yet to be finalised by the Department of Health. The table on the next page sets out the typical salaries (in 2005) of public sector doctors at different levels and stages of their careers.

Typical salaries and pay scales

POSITION	BASIC PAY	TOP PAY*	NOTES ON PAY
Hospital			
Foundation year one trainee	£19,703	£35,465	+ free hospital accommodation
Foundation year two+ trainee	£24,587	£50,191	Top pay would be after an additional three years' training
Specialist registrar	£27,483	£60,007	Top pay after three years in position plus basic specialist exams
Career grade doctor	£29,845	£72,892	Working directly with patients as a senior doctor
Consultant	£67,133	£90,838	May also receive up to £69,000 **extra** due to out-of-hours supplements and Clinical Excellence Awards
GP			
GP registrar (GPR)	Salary in last position held + a 65% supplement	£46,009 (typically)	For a GPR with three years' previous experience in a hospital post
Qualified GP	-	£71,588	For a self-employed, full-time GP

Source: NHS careers

These are 2005 figures. Figures for 2006 were not available when this guide was being prepared.

* Includes extra pay for out-of-hours work and pay banding to reflect intensity of different roles.

Case study

GP registrar

UMARAJINI KANNAN, 34

Route into medicine:

A levels in biology, mathematics and chemistry; BSc in biochemistry and chemistry at Queen Mary and Westfield College, London; medical degree at the University of Dundee

WHY MEDICINE?

After doing my first degree, I worked as a medical laboratory scientific officer at Lewisham Hospital. My work involved analysis and interpretation of blood specimens. My interest in these made me want to do a more challenging job in medicine that involved patient diagnosis.

WHY GENERAL PRACTICE?

After two years as a senior house officer, I did six months of care for the elderly, which I enjoyed, as you need to have a holistic approach to their management. I had originally planned to become a consultant in endocrinology, but trying to combine looking after a small child with working night shifts and weekends as a registrar in A&E was too difficult. So I investigated becoming a GP with an interest in other specialisms. I'd like to become a GP with a special interest in endocrinology, offering treatment in a practice context to patients with diabetes who would otherwise have to wait for a hospital appointment.

WHAT DOES YOUR CURRENT ROLE INVOLVE?

I work in the GP practice for two and a half days a week, plus a half-day tutorial with one of the practice GPs, when I can ask them about anything I want to know. I also spend half a day covering in a local nursing home and one day on a course for GP registrars in the Oxford Deanery. The final half-day is study leave, which I am spending on a hospital attachment, working in some specialisms I need to spend more time on.

THE BIGGEST CHALLENGES OF YOUR CAREER SO FAR?

Getting into medical school – both because I was already a graduate (there are only a limited number of places for graduate applicants) and because I hadn't done my GCSEs in the UK. Also, it's tough to combine work – and a daily commute from London to Oxfordshire – with raising a small child.

AND THE BEST BITS?

- Coming to work and seeing patients. Wonderful!
- Having supportive and well-informed colleagues and working in an up-to-date and well-run practice.
- In this practice, having immediate access to a day hospital, x-ray facilities and a range of other professionals such as physiotherapists.

UMA'S TOP TIPS

- Don't go into medicine unless you really want to do it. It needs hard work and commitment.
- When applying to medical school, talk to as many people as possible in the school to find out about the environment and facilities. For example, if you don't like urban environments, don't study in a big city.
- When you're called for interview, prepare very carefully and practise using specimen questions. If you can, make a visit in advance to the place where you've been called for interview and speak to the course tutors.

Which specialism?

With over 60 different specialist medical training programmes, there's something for everyone.

In theory, the range of programmes offers junior doctors a wealth of fields to choose from. In practice, however, many areas of medicine are very oversubscribed and competition to get in is very intense. Broadly speaking, the different hospital specialisms fall into two main groups: medical and surgical.

Medical work involves diagnosis and non-surgical treatments. Many of the specialities focus on particular organs, eg the heart (cardiology), or on disease, eg cancer (oncology).

Surgical work involves the in-theatre specialists, who operate on the body to address injury or disease.

However, some specialisms, like psychiatry and gynaecology, don't really sit in either of these two main groups. Examples of the most popular specialist fields, and what they involve, are outlined below.

EMERGENCY MEDICINE (FORMERLY ACCIDENT & EMERGENCY OR A&E)

The work:
Emergency services provide immediate care to the acutely ill and injured – ranging from major trauma and medical emergencies to a large volume of minor injuries and complaints.

The conditions:

The unpredictability of cases, the need to call on different medical knowledge from one case to another, the distress of patients, plus the demands of government waiting list targets all make this a pressurised environment, so you'll need nerves of steel.

The upside:

The opportunity to make a real, immediate difference to ease someone's pain, and working in the only place in the hospital that offers exposure to such a breadth of medicine.

The downside:

You may be exposed to patients with violent behaviour from drug or alcohol abuse, and there are also the potential demands of out-of-hours shift work.

For more info:

The College of Emergency Medicine
www.emergencymed.org.uk/cem.

OBSTETRICS & GYNAECOLOGY

The work:

Ranges from gynaecological oncology (eg treating cervical cancer), to treating menopause, to in vitro fertilisation (IVF), to foetal monitoring and even foetal surgery. On the obstetrics side, the doctor is responsible for the care of **two** patients simultaneously – mother and baby – spending a lot of time looking after women who are not ill but who are experiencing a major life event.

The conditions:

This is an area of work with extreme highs and lows, especially on the obstetrics side. You may also find yourself under pressure if you're the only specialist registrar capable of performing a caesarean section on a ward.

The upside:

It's one of the few fields that allow doctors to maintain an interest in both medicine and surgery.

The downside:

So much riding on successful results that can have a huge impact on an entire family.

For more info:

www.nhscareers.nhs.uk/nhs-knowledge_base/data/5464.html.

PSYCHIATRY

The work:

Mental illness is one of the biggest health problems in the UK. As the guardians of mental health, psychiatrists treat a whole range of medical conditions including depression, learning disabilities, eating disorders, drug and alcohol abuse, phobias and post-traumatic stress disorders, as well as helping people cope with emotional and stressful situations such as a bereavement or family trauma. It's an odd mix of intense one-to-one work and teamwork, as psychiatrists work closely in multidisciplinary teams with a variety of other healthcare professionals such as social workers. It is also possible to specialise in areas including child psychiatry and forensic psychiatry (ie working in a criminal or legal context, for example, treating and assessing offenders).

The conditions:

You could find yourself working in a variety of settings, such as care homes, secure psychiatric units, community centres and even prisons. It's also a field where flexible working options are readily accepted.

The upside:

If you're a 'people' person, psychiatry brings you directly into the very real human side of medicine and medical care.

The downside:

It can seem thankless, in that it can take a very long time to begin to see the effect of your work. In this field, remember that you're in it for the long haul.

For more info:

The Royal College of Psychiatrists
www.rcpsych.ac.uk.

RADIOLOGY

The work:

A radiologist focuses on the use of imaging to diagnose, treat and monitor disease. Ever-clearer imaging quality is creating more opportunities to offer image-guided treatment, sometimes without the need for surgical intervention. For this kind of work, the Royal College of Radiologists says a good knowledge of general medicine and surgery is paramount. The massive growth in applications of radiological imaging has resulted in a worldwide shortage of trained radiologists.

The conditions:

As most of the work is lab-based, doctors work individually and intensively on their own, and then interact with surgeons and specialists from numerous fields of medicine to give their findings and work out a treatment plan.

The upside:

Spotting disease early enough, thanks to attention to detail and improved image quality.

The downside:

Long, intense hours examining x-rays and scan results can be hard on eyesight.

For more info:

The Royal College of Radiologists
www.rcr.ac.uk.

SURGERY

The work:

In-theatre specialists spend their training years in general surgery and specialise as consultants in one or two fields: the fields could include reconstruction/ plastic, maxillofacial, colorectal and vascular surgery. Contrary to popular perception, surgeons do not spend the majority of their time in theatre. The average surgeon spends approximately one-and-a-half days per week in theatre, and the rest of their time on ward rounds and running outpatient clinics to follow up with patients.

The conditions:

Working conditions get easier as you go higher up the career ladder – but if you have a full theatre list, expect very early starts and long days.

The upside:

Surgery really suits the pragmatic and dynamic medic. You don't have to deal so much with the patient, and success (or failure) is more immediately apparent.

The downside:

There are fewer women at consultant surgeon level (just six per cent according to WIST – Women in Surgical Training, accessible via the Royal College of Surgeons).

For more info:

The Royal College of Surgeons (England)
www.rcseng.ac.uk.

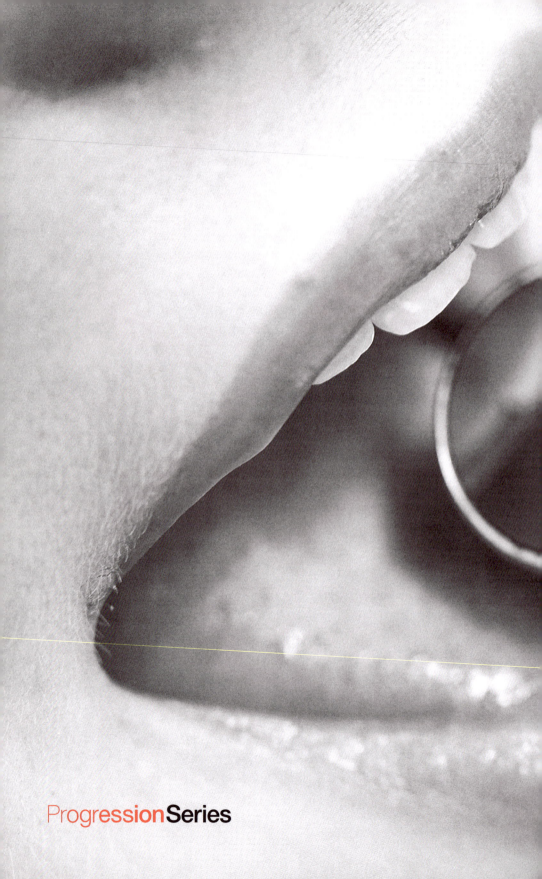

ProgressionSeries

Introducing dentistry

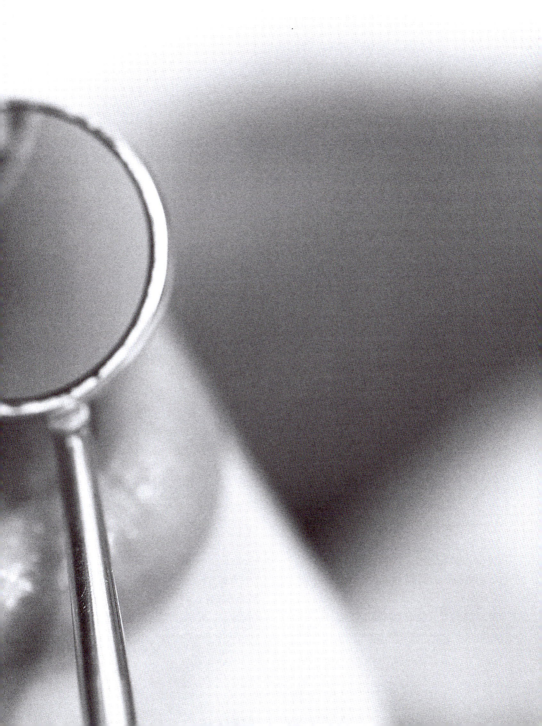

A career in dentistry

This section provides an overview of the main career choices, specialities, working conditions and pay for dentists in the UK today.

Compared to their medical colleagues, the majority of dental graduates have a much more straightforward career structure, since most dental students go into general dental practice. The number of dental specialities may be more limited, but those that exist are highly specialised.

GENERAL DENTAL PRACTITIONER

Most graduate dentists become general dental practitioners in public and (increasingly) private dental practices in local communities, treating all ages and all general dental complaints from fillings to extractions to bridges to crowns – and some cosmetic surgery.

Working conditions

Despite the pressures of dental emergencies and the limited resources from the NHS, general dental practitioners do usually have a high quality of life. They get to decide when, where and for how long they work. They start to earn a high salary quite soon after graduation; and they have a high degree of autonomy, especially if they run their own practice.

Pay

General dental practitioners are self-employed, and until April 2006, received a 'per item' fee from the NHS. But from April 2006 the system of payments to NHS dentists in England and Wales changed to one based on contracts. The amount of money paid to dentists under these contracts is based on an assessment of the typical amount of work done by the practice or practitioner over one year.

Typical salaries

POSITION	TYPICAL PAY*	NOTES ON PAY
Hospital		
Hospital dental services trainee	£24,587 – £34,477	Will be treated as the same grade of medical trainee
Specialist registrar	£27,483 – £44,733	A more advanced hospital trainee, by now working in a dental specialism
Dental consultant	£67,133 – £90,838	Leader of hospital dental team with relevant specialist qualifications
General Practice		
Vocational dental practitioner (VDP)	£26,520	A VDP is a trainee dentist in their first year of training after graduation
General dental practitioner (GDP)	£77,000 – £83,000	For a full-time, self-employed GDP, whose training is now complete
Community dental officer	£30,313 – £48,016	Unlike general dental practitioners, who are self-employed, community dental officers receive a salary

Source: NHS careers

* These are 2005 figures. Figures for 2006 were not available when this guide was being prepared.

Case study

Vocational dental practitioner

NICOLE MARRIOTT, 23

Route into medicine:

A levels in biology, chemistry, mathematics and general studies; dental degree at the University of Birmingham

WHY DENTISTRY?

My interest in a career in dentistry started when I had successful orthodontic treatment while growing up. When I did my work experience prior to entering the sixth form, I chose to spend it at the dental practice my family goes to, and really enjoyed it.

WHY GENERAL PRACTICE?

I really enjoy seeing a variety of cases and the people aspect is very important. In general practice you get to develop a wide range of skills. Because of this experience I feel confident that, no matter where I might work, I have the professional and social skills to treat any patient who might walk through the door. And the working hours in general practice are very accommodating – an important consideration if you need to combine work with, say, raising a family.

NICOLE'S TOP TIPS

- It's vital to get some first-hand experience of dentistry before you start to study.
- You need a high level of commitment to cope with the continuous studying and exams.
- Studying dentistry is expensive. Being good with money and able to budget really helps.
- Dentistry is very absorbing, so it's important to maintain outside interests.

WHAT DOES YOUR VOCATIONAL TRAINING INVOLVE?

I work in a purpose-built, award-winning practice in north-east Birmingham that deals mainly with NHS patients. There are four other associates, a hygienist and a community dentist. Every fortnight I go to the postgraduate centre in the City Hospital where I am able to exchange experiences with colleagues and peers, which is really useful. The vocational training year really introduces the business side of dentistry as, for example, when you're formulating a treatment plan for a patient, you have to be aware what everything will cost.

THE BIGGEST CHALLENGES OF YOUR TRAINING SO FAR?

Because dentistry is multidisciplinary, it's important to appreciate that every discipline you study during your course is of equal importance. Also, at the end of my fourth year, I wanted to do my elective study project in Barbados, making a comparison of general practice there and in the UK. I budgeted really carefully for the trip, but still needed additional funding from the dental school. Waiting for that money to come through was a very anxious time

AND THE BEST BITS?

- Getting feedback from satisfied patients. One patient told me that because of the treatment I had given her, she felt more confident about going for a job interview.
- Making some wonderful friends, who are now supportive colleagues.
- The excellent training at Birmingham Dental School.
- Looking forward to going to work in the morning!

Which specialism?

To specialise in dentistry mostly means you'll have to follow the hospital dentistry route. Once qualified, however, it is entirely possible and even common in some specialisms for the dental specialist to move out of the hospital setting to establish their own practice – for example, in orthodontics. The key dental specialisms are outlined below.

ORTHODONTICS

The work:

Orthodontics is the branch of dentistry concerned with growth of the face, development of the 'occlusion' (alignment of the upper and lower jaw) and the correction and prevention of occlusal abnormalities. These are the dental specialists responsible for that brace you might have worn as a child to correct overly protruding or badly aligned teeth.

The conditions:

Qualified orthodontists are likely to begin working in a specialist practice with more experienced colleagues, or may choose to establish a new practice (which is more complicated than setting up a general dental practice). They may provide treatment in the NHS or privately, or a mix of both. Hours of work will then be of their choosing and, like general dental practitioners, they will have a high-quality lifestyle with limited pressure.

The upside:

The opportunity for longer, more intricate, one-to-one treatments, and the satisfaction that comes from helping patients overcome conditions about which they are often self-conscious.

The downside:

Orthodontic treatments take time, so you'll need a lot of patience.

For more info:

The British Orthodontics Society www.bos.org.uk.

SPECIALITIES

Other 'dontics', dental specialities, include **periodontics** (treatment of gums), **endodontics** (treatment of the tooth root and surrounding tissue) and **prosthodontics** (replacement of missing teeth by prostheses). At present there is no special funding for trainees in these specialities, so the majority of trainees will be self-funding, and most will probably enter private practice.

For more information see:

British Society of Periodontology
www.bsperio.org

British Endodontic Society
www.britishendodonticsociety.org

British Prosthodontic Conference
www.bsrd.org.

ORAL AND MAXILLOFACIAL SURGERY

The work:

Nicknamed 'maxfax', this is a unique specialism in that surgeons must possess both a dental and a medical degree, as well as being on the Dental Register and having the requisite surgical qualifications. This specialty has its origins in wartime, when dental surgeons became prominent in devising local flap reconstruction of lost facial tissues. The core activity of the specialty is the management of facial trauma, both soft and hard tissue. However, approximately 80 per cent of mouth and jaw cancer is currently managed by this specialty, which also covers congenital abnormalities, such as a cleft palate.

The conditions:

'Maxfax' surgeons work in acute general hospitals, specialist hospitals and university teaching hospitals. They typically spend more time in theatre and on local anaesthesia operations than generalist surgeons. The work is a combination of emergencies and acute cases, plus follow-ups, or minor and aesthetic work carried out on an outpatient basis. The schedule for trainees also involves night and weekend 'on calls'.

The upside:

It has the most visible results of all surgery specialities – on the face.

The downside:

'Maxfax' has the longest, most demanding training requirements – starting with a dental and a medical degree.

For more info:

The British Association of Oral and Maxillofacial Surgeons www.baoms.org.uk.

SURGICAL DENTISTRY

The work:

This area of work deals with the diagnosis and surgical management of anomalies of the teeth and their supporting structures. In other words, surgical dentists work exclusively inside the mouth itself. Extracting wisdom teeth is a common procedure.

The conditions:

Treatment is normally carried out on an outpatient basis under local anaesthesia, so it's a more regular working day than for a 'maxfax' surgeon. Surgical dentists may also work in specialist practice, hospitals or a community dental service. If working in a hospital, they may be employed as associate specialists under the supervision of a consultant in oral and maxillofacial surgery and, as a result, may get to take on a wider clinical role.

The upside:

For those who still want to combine surgery with dentistry, the route to qualification is quicker than for maxillofacial surgery.

The downside:

Once you qualify, you'll still be restricted to working within the mouth and won't be able to work more widely on the head, face or neck.

For more info:

The British Association of Oral Surgeons www.baos.rcsed.ac.uk.

Case study

Specialist registrar in oral
and maxillofacial surgery

DEAN KISSUN, 39

Route into medicine:

A levels in biology, chemistry and physics; dental degree at the University of Manchester; medical degree at the University of Birmingham

WHY MEDICINE *AND* DENTISTRY?

When I was studying for my A levels, I went to an open day at King's College, London. One of the presentations was about oral and maxillofacial surgery – and that really started my interest. During the first year of my dental degree I saw a lot of oral surgery, and it struck me that this was the most interesting thing to do with a dental degree.

WHAT DOES BECOMING AN ORAL AND MAXILLOFACIAL SURGEON INVOLVE?

After graduating in dentistry, I was a general duties house officer at Manchester Dental Hospital, doing blocks of three to four months in different dental specialities. I then spent three more years in different hospitals before starting my medical degree. It isn't easy for people with dental degrees to get into medical school, and I was lucky that the people I was working for were very supportive and helped me prepare for the interview. It was a three-year course and because my

Fellowship in Dental Surgery (FDS)* had covered primary science, I had some flexibility with the exams. After graduating I became a house officer, spending six months in general surgery and six in general medicine. Then, as a senior house officer, I did rotations in orthopaedic, ENT and general surgery. In that time I passed my FRCS* exams which meant I could apply for my current position as a specialist registrar. I am now looking for a consultant post.

* FDS Fellowship in Dental Surgery: This was the principal postgraduate qualification awarded by the Royal College of Surgeons (RCS). The FDS has now been replaced by the MFDS (Membership of the Faculty of Dental Surgery).

* FRCS Fellow of the Royal College of Surgeons.

WHAT DOES AN ORAL AND MAXILLOFACIAL SURGEON DO?

I perform surgery for the management of facial injuries, head and neck cancers, salivary gland disorders, treatment of facial disproportion, jaw joint disorders, cysts and tumours of the jaw. I also do facial aesthetic surgery to help restore people's appearance after they have suffered a facial disfigurement. At the moment I am operating every day, treating emergency admissions involving facial fractures. One of the reasons I see so many cases of this kind is that my hospital, University Hospital Aintree, is one of just a few specialising in this kind of injury, so we take trauma cases from a wide catchment area with a population of 4 million.

THE BIGGEST CHALLENGE OF YOUR TRAINING SO FAR?

It's impossible to overestimate the time and financial commitments needed for this career pathway. And it's definitely not for people who want quick rewards. You need a great deal of inner motivation and self-belief.

AND THE BEST BITS?

- The great diversity of work within this specialty, both in the range of conditions we treat and in complexity – from very simple to very complex operations.
- Because people working in this area are so motivated, it tends to bring out the best in them and creates a stimulating working environment.
- Making a very visible difference to people's lives.
- Attending national and international meetings and learning from top people in the field.

DEAN'S TOP TIPS

- As well as having a career plan, it helps to have a life plan, so you can keep the two in balance.
- To work in this field you need to be able to meet a lot of targets and pass a lot of exams. It's not a good choice for people who aren't good at exams.
- The support and care of people close to you, who take an interest in your career, can make all the difference.

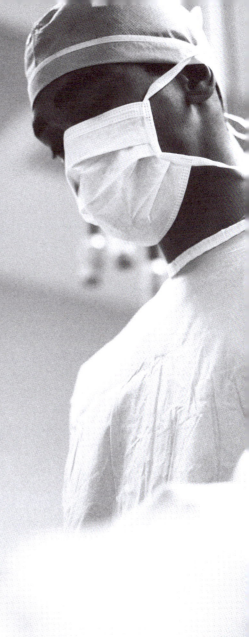

The career
for you?

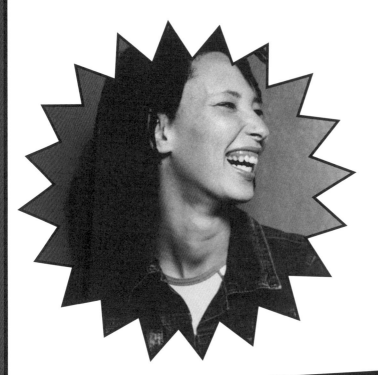
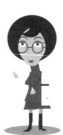

The career for you?

Being a successful doctor or dentist calls for more than an in-depth understanding of the relevant science. It also requires certain skills and personal qualities or 'attributes'.

To help you decide if a career in the medical or dental profession is for you, we suggest you consider the following questions:

- What do you want from your future work?
- What does the course typically involve?
- Which skills do doctors and dentists typically need?

WHAT DO YOU WANT FROM YOUR FUTURE WORK?

You may not have an instant answer for this now, but your current studies, work experience to date and even your hobbies can help give you clues about the kind of work you enjoy, and the skills you have already started to develop. Start with a blank sheet of paper and note down the answers to the questions we've provided below to help get you thinking. Be as brutally honest with yourself as you can. Don't write what you think will impress your teachers or parents; write what really matters to you and you'll start to see a pattern emerge.

ANSWERING THESE QUESTIONS MAY HELP YOU TO CHOOSE YOUR CAREER

- When you think of your future, in what kind of environment do you see yourself working? For example, office, outdoor, nine-to-five, high-pressure, regular routine.
- What are your favourite hobbies outside school?
- What is it about them you enjoy? For example, working with people, working out how things work.
- What are your favourite subjects in school?

- What is it about them that you enjoy most? For example, being able to create something, debating, problem solving, practical hands-on work.
- What do you dislike about the other subjects you're studying? (Writing 'the teacher' doesn't count!)
- Which aspects of your work experience have you most enjoyed?

WHAT DOES THE COURSE TYPICALLY INVOLVE?

Course intensity: It's especially important for medical students to know that the first stage of your studies – the undergraduate degree – will require great stamina, as it's typically five years of intensive studying for exams, plus numerous in-hospital placements or 'rotations'. So if you don't see yourself spending hours studying when your friends on other courses have long since left for the day or the weekend, or have even completed their course and are off earning money, then maybe medicine is not for you. Would-be dentists should also know that much of the course is now chemistry-based (you'll study biochemistry), as well as the more expected courses on anatomy, physiology and pathology, and dental materials science.

Course structure: All courses are a combination of '**academic**' (ie studying sciences) work and '**clinical**' (ie hands-on, in-hospital or clinics) work. Most universities now mix the two. But others (most notably Oxford and Cambridge) split the course, with the first two to three years spent in the classroom and on lecture-based 'academic' work, studying sciences, and the latter two to three years spent on placements or 'rotations' in hospitals.

In addition, some medical and dental schools are increasing the amount of '**self-directed**' learning (where students are given a task, a list of objectives, and told to go away and research it, then come back to discuss what they've found out).

Some courses also offer an '**intercalated**' degree, ie the chance to take one to two years out to study another science-related subject in the middle of your medical or dental degree. This is of most value to students who identify early on that they want to specialise, particularly in a research field.

It's important to find out how much of the course teaching is lecture-based, self-directed and hands-on, and if it offers an 'intercalated' option

WHICH SKILLS DO DOCTORS AND DENTISTS TYPICALLY NEED?

Without doubt, admissions tutors for both medicine and dentistry look for **strong academic ability**, just to prove your ability to cope with the straight science, plus clear **evidence of a commitment to medicine or dentistry** as a career (which can usually be demonstrated via work experience placements). Beyond this, the following key skills are required of any potential medical or dental student.

- Excellent communication skills – speaking and listening – to be able to explain complicated medical jargon in ordinary language, and to draw out crucial information from patients, often when they're under stress, and to put patients at their ease.
- Empathy, ie a degree of sensitivity and understanding of each patient's situation and feelings; dentists, in particular, need to have strong 'people' skills, as you'll be providing dental care for people of all ages and you'll be seeing them on an ongoing basis.
- Problem-solving ability, ie the ability quickly to assess and analyse a situation or 'case'.
- Attention to detail – the ability to pick up on the smallest of signs or symptoms.
- Calmness under fire – mostly for hospital doctors. Given the combination of long hours and unpredictability of cases, you've got to be able to cope under pressure.
- Confidentiality – knowing what to communicate, when and to whom.
- Stamina – to cope with the 12-hour shifts and the on-call work.
- Decisiveness – to be able to back your own judgement and make decisions under fire.

And, of course, it helps if you can stand the sight of blood, and have a steady hand if you're thinking of surgery…!

Case study

Trainee doctor
(foundation year two)

SYED ARSALAN RAZA, 27

Route into medicine:
Higher secondary school exams in Pakistan in biology, chemistry, physics and English; medical degree at the University of Karachi; clinical internship in Karachi followed by research post

WHY MEDICINE?

Seeing my father being treated by good, caring doctors in hospital was an inspiration to me. And my parents were keen for me to go into medicine. I also wanted to do a job in which I could serve people and share their problems.

WHAT DOES YOUR CURRENT TRAINING INVOLVE?

F2 is a pilot programme at the moment. The concept of foundation is to have a mix of specialities that don't necessarily have a close relationship to each other. I'm doing a rotation of one year in three specialisms. I'm currently doing cardiology, having already done neonatology (working with new-born babies). My next rotation will be neurology. I would like to specialise in radiology.

WHY RADIOLOGY?

Because the basics of the specialism involve interpreting images, radiology is thought of as being rather isolated from patients. But I think it's the most progressive field in medicine at the moment. Increasingly, radiologists are involved in clinical care and patient contact, for example, when doing an ultrasound scan or a procedure such as taking a tissue sample. There's so much to learn in radiology that you acquire new skills and are faced with new challenges every day.

THE BIGGEST CHALLENGE OF YOUR COURSE SO FAR?

When you start at medical college, you concentrate on the theoretical basics and are likely to be deficient in practical skills. But as you start to acquire those skills you have less time to study the theory, even though you need to keep up to date with new developments. So keeping theory and practice in balance is a challenge. In this respect, continuing professional development (which is part of the training here in the Oxford Radcliffe Hospitals and involves courses, lectures and study days) is very useful.

AND THE BEST BITS?

- The satisfaction of seeing patients get better and regain their energy and interest in life.
- Passing exams. It's always a relief to get one out of the way!
- Being in Oxford. And the atmosphere in the John Radcliffe Hospital, which is friendly as well as academic.

SYED'S TOP TIPS

- Coming from overseas makes it doubly difficult to get a hospital post. When I first arrived, I did an attachment without pay to learn how the system works before I began applying for jobs.
- Being a doctor means sharing your life with your patients and sometimes having to give them priority. Knowing this from the outset makes this aspect of the job easier to accept.
- Hard work is the key to success. You might be excused for not being extremely bright, but never for being lazy.
- It's very important to make time in your life for social activities – even though this can be difficult when you're working unsocial hours.

Alternative careers

Ilf the traditional doctor or dentist roles don't feel quite 'you', but you still have a strong leaning towards science, there are many roles in the medical and dental fields to choose from.

Below are some of the main related professions.

ALLIED HEALTH PROFESSIONS

These are the 70,000 professionals who work alongside doctors and dentists mostly for the physical rehabilitation and revival of patients, eg physiotherapists, speech and language therapists, paramedics, dieticians. Each allied health profession has its own entry requirements and path to qualification. It is possible to enter most of these professions at different levels. For example, if you don't have A levels, but do have four or five good GCSEs, you could join in a support or 'therapy assistant' role.

See www.nhscareers.nhs.uk.

HEALTHCARE SCIENTISTS

Biomedical scientists carry out lab tests to support doctors in diagnosing and treating disease. The majority specialise in a particular area, eg pharmacy or histopathology (the analysis of tissue samples from surgical ops).

You can become a biomedical scientist via several routes:

- take a degree in biomedical science
- take a degree in another science, then take a 'top-up' course
- go in after A levels, in which case you'll still have to take a biomed degree on day release.

It's also possible, and in many cases preferable, to move into research and lab work after you've qualified with a medical degree. In fact, some fields are closed to non-medical graduates. Check with the Institute of Biomedical Science www.ibms.org.

Pharmacists (in hospitals or in the community) make up prescriptions, monitor dosages and advise on use of medication. The route to becoming a pharmacist is more straightforward – you've got to do a four-year Master of Pharmacy degree followed by one year of training based in a pharmacy practice.

See Royal Pharmaceutical Society of Great Britain www.rpsgb.org.uk.

DENTAL HYGIENIST AND DENTAL THERAPIST

A dental hygienist works to prevent dental problems from arising by performing routine 'hygiene' including scaling and polishing teeth, applying sealants and advising on oral hygiene. You'll need two A levels and the General Dental Council's Diploma in Dental Hygiene.

See British Dental Hygienists' Association www.bdha.org.uk.

Dental therapists can do all of the above and more – including taking dental impressions, dental radiography, placing preformed crowns and even doing extractions under certain conditions. You'll need two A levels and a Diploma in Dental Therapy (which takes 27 months).

See British Association of Dental Therapists www.badt.org.uk.

DENTAL TECHNICIAN

This is the unseen and unsung hero or heroine of the dental world, who sits in a lab making the dentures, crowns, veneers, bridges and dental braces on which the dentist and the patient rely. Your 'customers' are the dentists, and you'll work to their orders and prescriptions, using a range of materials, for example, gold, porcelain and plastic, to design and build appliances to meet each patient's need. The entry requirement is a BTEC National Diploma in Dental Technology, for which A levels are more than enough for entry.

See British Dental Technicians' Association www.dta-uk.org.

MEDICAL JOURNALISM

This is a very fast-growing field, and an option for those who decide they'd rather observe their profession and use their medical knowledge to educate the wider public, some of whom may be confused by medical jargon and processes. Some universities now offer degrees in medical journalism, in some cases open only to medical undergraduates who have completed their pre-clinical years.

See Medical Journalists' Association www.mja-uk.org.

Case study

Consultant paediatric
and vascular anaesthetist

JOSIE BROWN, 44

Route into medicine:

A levels; medical degree at the University of Newcastle upon Tyne; 11 years' relevant medical exams and training at a variety of hospitals in the UK, and a year in Australia working in anaesthesia and neonatal intensive care

WHY MEDICINE?

I had planned to become a psychiatrist. But studying psychiatry as a medical undergraduate made me realise it wasn't for me! I was always interested in doing something that would contribute to society and help people.

WHY ANAESTHETICS?

You get the opportunity to work independently at an early stage. I also like the fact that things can happen very fast in the operating theatre – if you administer an injection, it takes 30 seconds to work, so you have instant feedback! I went into paediatric anaesthesia because I really enjoy working with children. It's technically challenging because things happen even faster with children than they do with adults as their metabolism and circulation work more quickly.

It's unusual to combine vascular anaesthesia with paediatric work, but vascular offers an interesting and challenging contrast – as you tend to deal with many more patients who are critically ill, it really maintains your skills.

WHAT DOES YOUR CURRENT ROLE INVOLVE?

I first see patients on the ward. When they go into theatre I give them an anaesthetic and then look after them throughout surgery, continuously monitoring circulation, breathing, temperature, depth of anaesthesia and so on. I bring them round immediately afterwards and later see if they need more pain relief.

I also do a range of administrative and teaching work. An interesting project I'm working on at the moment is for the Royal College of Anaesthetists. I'm a member of a team developing information to be given to children who will be undergoing anaesthesia. One of the challenges is to work out how best to communicate this information. It will probably involve computers or games.

THE BIGGEST CHALLENGES OF YOUR CAREER SO FAR?

Initially, surviving the training and the hours – and the tough examinations. There is also a considerable level of responsibility in anaesthesia – and the possibility of a patient coming to serious harm either because of my actions or those of someone I might be supervising. Also, in my particular area of anaesthetics, one of the greatest challenges is providing anaesthesia to premature babies, who might weigh as little as 500 grams. In such cases you have to work really hard to maintain breathing and circulation.

AND THE BEST BITS?

- Seeing people waking up comfortable and pain free after major surgery.
- The close relationships you develop with colleagues in the theatre team.
- The parties!

JOSIE'S TOP TIPS

- When thinking of applying to do medicine, don't just consider the academic components. I didn't get into medical school when I first applied, so I worked for a year as a care assistant in a residential home for the elderly. That experience helped enormously when I reapplied – and has also been a tremendous influence on the way I work.
- You need a good level of self-reliance and self-confidence in this job, as you need to give advice in a way that carries weight and reflects self-belief.
- Manual dexterity is important for performing procedures.
- In anaesthetics you need to be comfortable dealing with equipment. An A level in physics can be useful.

Entry routes

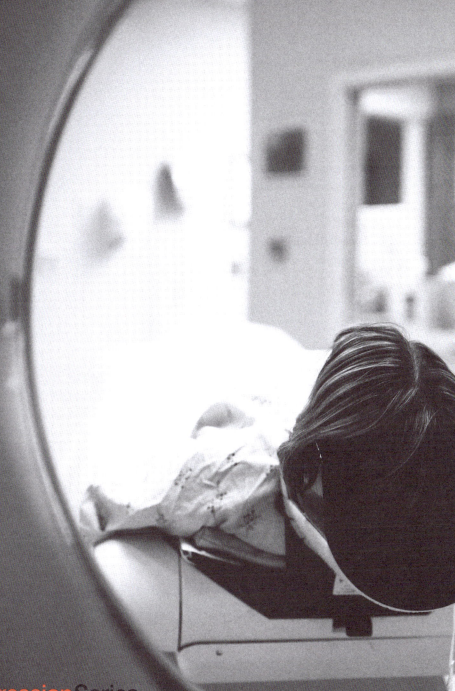

Routes to qualification

MEDICINE – NEW FOUNDATION PROGRAMME

Introduced in August 2005, the foundation programme is the new training framework for postgraduate medical education in the UK. The first year of post medical school training is now known as F1, and the second year as F2. For new medical graduates, the foundation programme aims to offer a coherent, managed programme of learning integrated into trainees' first introduction into working in the NHS. A commitment to improved career planning for doctors early in their careers means that you will have a better understanding of the breadth of career opportunities in the NHS, access to good information about future workforce trends in clinical specialities and – most importantly – the opportunity to think about and discuss your own attributes and aspirations and align these to the likelihood of success.

The later part of the foundation programme is still being introduced, but in essence, qualifying as a hospital doctor or GP will involve three main stages:
1 Medical degree +
2 Generalist training, known as the Foundation Programme +
3 Specialist training, including specialist exams.

The chart opposite outlines the main stages, and how long they will take.

FROM MEDICAL STUDENT TO SENIOR HOSPITAL DOCTOR OR GP

9-15 years total

1 MEDICAL DEGREE

Five years

Covers basic medical sciences and practical clinical activities, and gives students exposure to the different specialities within medicine.

2A F1 TRAINEE

One year

The first year of Foundation Programme training, involving basic in-hospital training under supervision. F1 training will typically involve a number of rotations, including general medicine and general surgery. There will also be formal teaching. You should be allocated an F1 posting by your medical school. Successful completion of the F1 year will result in full registration with the General Medical Council (GMC).

2B F2 TRAINEE

One year

More generalist training, involving at least one attachment allowing experience in acute care, plus formal teaching and a supervised audit project.

3 SPECIALIST TRAINING (RUN-THROUGH TRAINING)

- Approximately five to six years.
- You will now move into a specialist field.
- Hospital training will typically lead to a certificate of specialist training and consultant status.

3 GENERAL PRACTICE TRAINING (RUN-THROUGH TRAINING)

- Approximately three years.
- This part of your training will probably be community-based and you'll still have to sit the general practice specialism exams.

CERTIFICATE OF COMPLETION OF TRAINING (CCT)

CONSULTANT

GP PRINCIPAL

Qualifying will take longer if:

- **you take an 'intercalated' course** – ie an undergraduate course sandwiched around another year's (or two years') study of a related subject, for example, biomedicine, microbiology. If you're interested in this option, you should ask the medical schools if it is offered before you apply
- **you have to take a pre-med course** – ie you don't have the necessary science A levels, so you take a 30-week pre-med course to bring you up to A level standard
- **you work 'flexibly' while completing your training** – ie you work part-time or job share or take a career break part-way through.

QUALIFYING IN NORTHERN IRELAND AND SCOTLAND

Entry requirements, course content and career paths are the same all across the UK. Scottish Highers are acceptable at medical and dental schools throughout the UK, in which case mostly A and B grades will be preferred.

Case study

Sixth-year medical student

MARK HOHENBERG, 24

Route into medicine:

A levels in biology, chemistry and maths; medical degree at Royal Free and University College Medical School (London)

WHY MEDICINE?

I've always looked for a challenge. And around the time I was making decisions about my career, I was really starting to enjoy biology, so medicine was an obvious choice. During my gap year I did a four-month placement in Southern India, working closely alongside a hospital doctor. That confirmed for me that I'd made the right choice.

*NGO Non-governmental organisation: eg Médecins sans Frontières.

IN WHICH AREA WOULD YOU LIKE TO SPECIALISE?

It's still too early for me to be 100 per cent certain. I love variety and I also like to travel, so somewhere down the line I would like to work for an NGO* or perhaps the World Health Organisation. My top choice of specialism at the moment is international health (public health and epidemiology) – for which I have an excellent mentor, although other possibilities are psychiatry or infectious diseases. Ideally I'd like to find a way to combine a policy role with practising clinical medicine.

THE BIGGEST CHALLENGES OF YOUR STUDIES SO FAR?

Finding the right balance between work and social life. Doctors like to go out and have a good time, but when you start to do clinical medicine, you also have to consider your responsibility to patients.

Maintaining interests outside your studies – and outside medicine – won't only help your career prospects, but will also help you develop as a person. You'll be a better doctor and colleague for it. I've been principal of the Royal Society of Medicine student members' group, for example, representing 890 students. I also do a lot of sport, especially rowing.

Also, it can be hard to study and make enough money to survive, particularly when you start clinical medicine. Your grades can suffer if you try to work throughout your degree. And you'll find you really need your weekends!

AND THE BEST BITS?

- The friends – people you'll meet from all walks of life, who will be a close part of your life for six years, and hopefully beyond.
- The pre-clinical years. They're not as hard as what comes later, and are a good chance to enjoy university life to the full (and meet non-medics!)
- My final-year elective in the Solomon Islands, working in a hospital covering a huge area. I was effectively working as a junior doctor and at one point was even left in charge of the hospital! It was the best place I've ever visited and the best part of my medical life so far.

MARK'S TOP TIPS

- Get as much experience within medicine as possible before deciding to enter it full time. It has to be what **you** want to do.
- Take a gap year if you can. It's much harder to take time out to see the world once you're a doctor.
- Go into university with an open mind. You will have fun, and you will meet new people and have new experiences. Take advantage of everything you can learn from your lecturers.
- Get a diary and use it. Good time management is probably one of the most important skills for a doctor.

Routes to qualification

DENTISTRY

Qualifying as a General Dental Practitioner involves two main stages:

1 Dental degree +
2 one year's professional in-practice training.

Qualifying as a hospital dental specialist takes longer, but also requires two stages:

1 Dental degree +
2 several years' specialist in-hospital training, including specialist exams.

Qualifying as a dental surgeon (ie oral or maxillofacial) takes longer again, and requires three stages:

1 Dental degree +
2 several years' specialist in-hospital training, including specialist exams +
3 the small matter of a medical degree, which you'll probably take while training.

The following diagram shows the key qualification stages.

FROM DENTAL STUDENT TO GENERAL PRACTITIONER OR EVEN DENTAL SURGEON

1 DENTAL DEGREE

Five years

Covers basic medical sciences, anatomy, pathology, physiology and practical clinical activities, plus dental science materials.

▼ ▼ ▼

For general dental practitioners

For non-surgical hospital-based specialisms

For dental surgery specialism

2 VOCATIONAL DENTAL PRACTITIONER

One year

This training usually involves working under supervision on your own patient list in a general dental practice.

2 F1 OR F2 TRAINEE

Approximately two years

You'll have to join the new 'Foundation' medical trainee route and start to gain general experience of a range of hospital specialities, before you can start to focus on your preferred dental speciality.

3 MEDICAL DEGREE

Approximately four years

Those wishing to become dental surgeons will have to qualify in medicine either before or during their specialist hospital training.

▼ ▼

GENERAL DENTAL PRACTITIONER

One year

At first you'll probably work as an 'associate' practitioner in someone else's practice, and will pay part of the fees you earn to the practice owner in return for use of the surgery, equipment and staff. Later on, you may become a practice owner (principal).

'RUN-THROUGH GRADES'

Approximately five years

You'll now be working in one or two dental specialisms. By the end of this stage you should have completed the exams for the specialism you've chosen.

▼

DENTAL SPECIALIST

For example, orthodontist, periodontist, oral surgeon.

6-15+ years total

Case study

Fifth-year dental student

Route into dentistry:

A levels in English, history and maths; pre-medical/pre-dental course* followed by dental degree at the University of Manchester

WHY DENTISTRY?

I worked as a dental nurse to fund my gap year work experience in Kenya. After a few months I could see how much job satisfaction dentistry offered and decided to train to become a dentist even though I hadn't done science A levels. At that point I started to research foundation courses.

*pre-medical/pre-dental course: A conversion course to the sciences for students with arts A levels

WHAT HAS YOUR DEGREE COURSE COVERED SO FAR?

Two years of pre-clinical academic study focused on problem-based learning, where we worked in groups to research a specific case or problem and reach a conclusion about it, with a tutor on hand to make sure we didn't miss anything important. In year 3 we began by making dentures, then learned clinical skills – working on 'phantom heads' and learning how to sit, use instruments and so on, gradually progressing to more complex clinical techniques. In this final year we're learning to make clinical decisions and draw up treatment plans. Along the way I've also done outreach programmes – spending half a day a week for 15 weeks in a particular dental service or specialist clinic.

IN WHICH AREA WOULD YOU LIKE TO SPECIALISE?

After my vocational training year, I would like to go back into a hospital to do my general professional training (GPT) followed by my professional exams. I'm keeping an open mind at the moment about my options, but having really enjoyed my work experience last summer in a maxillofacial unit in Brighton, I'm planning to apply to a similar unit in my second GPT year. But it's possible along the way that I will discover that I love general practice and decide to opt for that!

THE BIGGEST CHALLENGE OF YOUR COURSE SO FAR?

The change from performing a treatment plan mapped out by someone else, to getting in a patient from scratch, diagnosing their problem and drawing up and implementing an appropriate plan. The challenge is to give treatment that doesn't just work then and there, but will prove over time to have been the right choice.

AND THE BEST BITS?

- An outreach programme in a personal dental service, treating adult patients in a general practice setting. More realistic and enjoyable than treating cases in a dental hospital, where patients tend to be used to being treated by students.
- Learning how to treat children. It's challenging and rewarding.
- Oral surgery. I loved taking out my first tooth! I find the range of work involved in extractions really interesting.

RUPERT'S TOP TIPS

- Visit a dentist and get some work experience before you apply to dental school, so you can see what it's like to do the job.
- Teamwork and communication are very important in dentistry. You're likely to be better at these if you're a well-rounded person, so keep up your other interests.
- You don't have to follow the science route at school to become a dentist.

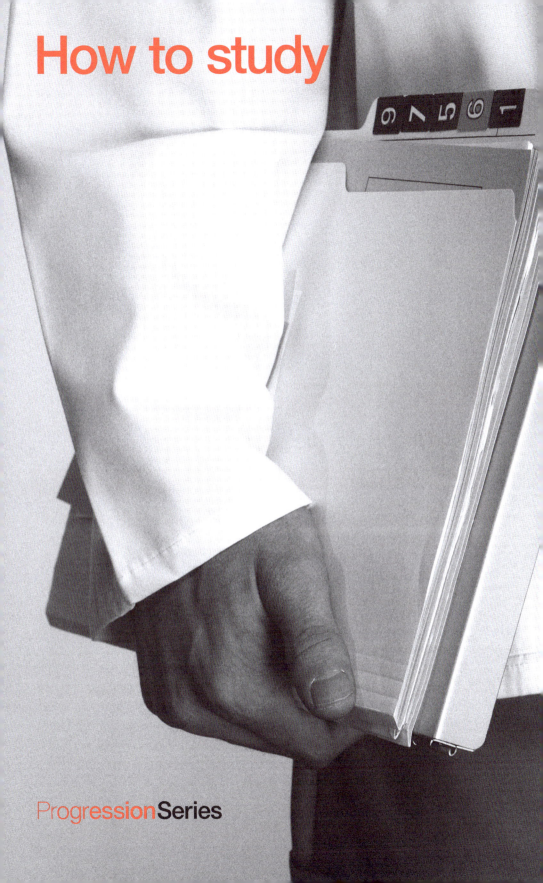

How to study

How to study

ENTRY REQUIREMENTS

Which subjects?

Contrary to popular belief, you no longer have to have all three sciences at A level to get into medical school. What's more, chemistry, not biology, is the most important subject at A level for entry to most medical schools.

However, the jury's still out on the need for biology at A level as well. Critics claim that students who don't have biology A level are at a disadvantage in the first year of med school, which is highly science-based. But once students enter the more clinical (ie practical) side of the course, the gap is closed.

HOW DO I FIND THE BEST COURSE FOR ME?

For courses on offer, see 'Course Search' at ucas.com.

Download a copy of the joint UCAS/QAA (Quality Assurance Agency for Higher Education) publication *How do I find the best course for me?* from ucas.com/getting/before/qaa.pdf. This provides some critical questions to ask before choosing higher education.

Applicants are advised to use various sources of information in order to make their choices for higher education, including the Course Search facility and Stamford Test at ucas.com. League tables might be a component of this research, but applicants should bear in mind that these tables attempt to rank institutions in an overall order, which reflects the interests, preoccupations and decisions of those who have produced and edited them. The ways in which they are compiled vary greatly and you need to look closely at the criteria that have been used. Applicants can also order hard copies of *How do I find the best course for me?* from UCAS Publication Services on 01242 544610, for additional information on choosing courses in higher education.

Which grades?

Competition for places in UK medical schools is very intense – reportedly six applications for every medical school place – so straight As or AAB at A level is a common entry grade requirement for the leading medical schools today. Certainly an A in chemistry is a great start, but most medical schools will look for high grades in at least one, more likely two, sciences at A level, plus another strong, academic subject. General studies is not considered a valid A level by medical schools. Increasingly, medical schools are also taking GCSE grades into account as another way to filter the growing number of straight A students.

What if you don't have any science A levels?

In theory, NHS Careers says you can still apply, but in practice, given the already stiff competition among students with science A levels, your odds are not great. The good news, however, is that a number of universities now offer 'pre-medical' and 'pre-dental' courses precisely for students with non-science A levels. These 'pre-' courses typically last 30 weeks and are designed to bring non-science students up to A level standard in the three sciences.

TOP TIP

Don't be afraid to pick up the phone – university admissions offices welcome enquiries directly from students, rather than careers officers on your behalf. It shows you're genuinely interested and committed to your own career early on.

Finding a course

There are a limited number of medicine and dentistry courses available in higher education in the UK. Moreover, it is a popular career choice and competition is fierce. How do you find out more information to make an informed decision?

Our advice to you is to do some careful research and seek guidance on your choice of university or college and course. Your teachers or careers advisers or the universities and colleges themselves can provide useful guidance. But the decision you need to make on high-demand courses, such as those you are applying for, is whether you are flexible about your choice of career. If you perform well on another course, it might be possible to gain entry to a four-year graduate medicine course. The other route, if you are determined to follow your original choice, is to consider taking a gap year and reapplying. Whatever route you choose, the best advice is to ensure you gain the highest grades possible. The better your performance, the wider your options will be.

Once you've made a list of the courses you are interested in, read the university entry profiles (see the next page) to find out what particular courses offer. You can then follow this up by looking at university department websites and generally finding out as much as you can about the course, department and university. Don't be afraid to contact them to ask for more information, request their prospectus or arrange an open day visit.

UCAS WEBSITE – UCAS.COM

Whether you want advice about applying to higher education, to check out what courses are available, to find out what qualifications you need, or to monitor the status of your application, ucas.com is THE place to start. The UCAS website is one of the most popular websites in the UK and the most heavily used educational one, with over 50 million page impressions a month. It is popular for good reason. From it, you can use Course Search as a quick and easy way to find out more about the courses you are interested in, including the vital code information you will need to include in your application later on. From Course Search, you can link to the websites of the universities and colleges in the UCAS system. Once you've applied through UCAS, you can use Track to check the progress of your application, including any decisions from universities or colleges, and you can make decisions online. You can check progress using your mobile phone if it's WAP-enabled.

Entry profiles

WHAT ARE THEY?

Entry profiles give potential applicants to higher education specific information to help them make informed decisions about the courses they apply for. Detailed knowledge about the course, formal entry requirements and the qualities and experiences institutions are looking for in their applicants can help ensure that every applicant finds their way onto the right course. Entry profiles are published on the UCAS website and can be reached using Course Search. So they are available for all potential applicants and their advisers to see as they start making important decisions about where to apply. All course providers are asked to contribute entry profiles for the UCAS website and a selection also appears in this book.

WHY USE THEM?

Courses can vary enormously at different universities and colleges. Differences in course content, structure, optional modules, and the department's approach to teaching and learning can make the experience of studying a particular subject different for students at different institutions, even before the size and location of the institution are taken into account.

It is important that you are fully informed about the courses and the institutions offering them before you apply, and know what qualities are being sought in an applicant. Then you can avoid mistakes and make fully informed choices.

HOW DO I USE THE ENTRY PROFILES?

▪ When you find courses that interest you, you can
read some of the entry profiles in this book or search
for the entry profile via Course Search at ucas.com.
Look for the symbol EP after the course title on the
results page. This tells you that it has a complete
entry profile.

▪ Courses without the EP symbol have qualification
details only.

▪ When you click on the course title, you will be taken
through to the course information you will need to
complete your application. You will find the entry
profile link immediately below this information. This
link will take you to the entry profile for this course.

Choosing your institution

People look for different things from their university course, but the checklist opposite sets out the kinds of factors all prospective students should consider when choosing their university. Enjoy your course – and good luck in your chosen career!

WHAT TO CONSIDER WHEN CHOOSING YOUR MEDICINE OR DENTISTRY COURSE

Grades required	Check out the university website or prospectus, or call up the medical/dental school admissions office. Some universities specify 'grades' required, eg AAB, while others specify 'points' required, eg 340. If they ask for points, it means they're using the UCAS 'tariff' system, which basically awards points to different types and levels of qualification. For example, an A grade at A level = 120 points; a B grade at A level = 100 points, etc. The full tariff table is available at www.ucas.com.
University location	Do you want to stay close to home? Do you want a city or campus university?
University 'ethos'	Find out if the medical/dental school is linked to a 'teaching hospital' – which should mean the hospital where you spend your rotations will be more oriented towards (ie have more time for) medical students.
Prospects	You generally get your first medical job in a hospital linked to the university, for example, in one of the hospitals where you spent a rotation, so find out which hospitals have links with each medical school.
Cost	Ask the admissions office about top-up fees and financial assistance. (After your further year as a med student, your fees will be paid for you.)
Degree type	Do you want a 'traditional' course, ie teaching science during the first one to two years, and then three years 'clinical' training in a hospital; or an 'integrated' course, ie the 'science' and the 'clinical' stages inter-mixed, so you start your rotations earlier on?
Facilities for medical/ dental students	Find out, for example, if there's a careers adviser dedicated to medical and dental students, or if there's a medical placements officer, who takes charge of matching students to rotations.
'Fit'	Even if all the above criteria stack up, this one relies on gut feel – go and visit the medical school if you can, and see if it's 'you'.

Case study

Trainee doctor
(foundation year two)

EDWARD HYDE, 24

Route into medicine:
A levels in biology, chemistry, physics, general studies; medical degree at the University of Bristol

WHY MEDICINE?

I love working with people. I don't like being bored, so I wanted to work in an area that would challenge me and where I could learn on the job. I wanted to do something scientific and be able to make a difference.

HOW DID YOU DECIDE WHICH COURSE TO CHOOSE?

Coming from South Devon, I wanted somewhere reasonably close to home. I didn't want to be stuck in a lab doing something purely science-based, so I looked for a course with a more integrated approach and

plenty of patient contact. In fact, this aspect of the course has increased still further since I did it. I also liked Bristol as a place, which was very important since I was going to spend several years there.

IN WHICH AREA OF MEDICINE WOULD YOU LIKE TO SPECIALISE?

I'm planning to do obstetrics and gynaecology, which is a bit unusual these days. One reason seems to be that many students don't have positive experiences in this specialism. It can be surprisingly difficult to attend live

ED'S TOP TIPS

- Medicine is a lifestyle choice. Try to get as much work experience as you can, so you really understand what you're getting yourself into.
- Apply to a university in a place you like.
- If you really want to do medicine, persevere. At school there were plenty of people who were pessimistic about me getting into this. I worked really hard and proved them wrong.
- Always keep a positive attitude and learn from your mistakes

deliveries of babies if you're a non-midwife, a student and male! I had never thought of doing this specialism, but then I spent some time doing obstetrics at Taunton Hospital and it was a real eye-opener. I found everything about the experience really interesting and was hooked from then on. I also did an obstetrics and gynaecology elective in New Zealand in my fifth year and probably got more hands-on experience than I would have done in the UK. I also like the fact that the specialism contains a good mix of medicine and surgery.

THE BIGGEST CHALLENGE OF YOUR TRAINING SO FAR?

My first weekend on call. On the Saturday morning I was confronted with an extremely sick patient and the knowledge that it was down to me to decide what to do. I did what I could, then called for senior help – which was exactly the right thing to do. Nowadays I handle that kind of situation regularly on my own.

AND THE BEST BITS?

- Making a difference. For example, knowing that by making the right intervention at the right time to stop something getting worse, I've improved a patient's long-term survival prospects.
- The people you work with. They can make all the difference when you've got a horrid job to do.
- The intellectual challenge, and learning new things. And realising how far I've come since I was a student.

How will they choose you?

ADMISSIONS TESTS

Students applying to some courses are required to sit an admissions test as part of the application process. Details follow of some of the medicine and dentistry courses that use admissions tests as part of their selection criteria. This is not a definitive list, so check with the university or college for the most up-to-date information on their admissions tests. A list of tests can be found on www.ucas.com/tests/index.html.

Admissions tests are a way to manage application numbers for high-demand courses by helping to differentiate fairly between well-qualified applicants. They can widen access and participation in higher education as they measure academic potential without being influenced by educational background.

Admissions tests broaden and complement other selection criteria as they often assess aptitude and reasoning rather than achievement and recall.

Admissions tests do not generally require additional teaching, although applicants should familiarise themselves with a specimen paper beforehand. Check with the test centre about what type of preparation is required. It is usually the applicant's own responsibility to ensure they are entered for a test by the closing date. Some tests are taken at the applicant's school or college, others require applicants to sit the test at a test centre or at the university or college as part of an interview day. Overseas applicants may not be required to sit an admissions test (see page 85) – check with the course provider.

These tests are being used for medicine and
dentistry courses.

- BioMedical Admissions Test (BMAT) (see next page).
- Graduate Medical School Admissions
  Test (GAMSAT) (see page 72).
- Medical School Admissions Test (MSAT) (see page 74).
- UK Clinical Aptitude Test (UKCAT) (see page 76).

The 'BMAT'

BioMedical Admissions Test

WHICH UNIVERSITIES REQUIRE IT?

Currently three of the top UK universities (others also require it for entry to veterinary studies):

- University of Cambridge
- Imperial College London (University of London)
- University of Oxford
- University College London (University of London).

WHAT DOES IT INVOLVE?

A written test under exam conditions, comprising these three sections.

- 60 minutes, multi-choice questionnaire to assess your 'aptitude and skills', ie how good you are at analysing and interpreting data.

- 30 minutes, multi-choice paper to test your scientific knowledge in biology, chemistry, physics and maths.
- 30 minutes, written task, eg essay on a choice of topics.

WHERE IS THE TEST HELD?

At one of several BMAT-approved test centres around the UK.

WHEN IS IT HELD?

Once a year, usually in early November.

HOW CAN I REGISTER FOR THE TEST?

With the test centre direct. To find a test centre, go to the BMAT website and click on the 'How I register' section on the left navigation bar.

HOW MUCH DOES IT COST?

For candidates within the UK, the cost is £26. The closing date for entries for 2006 is Friday 29 September 2006.

HOW CAN I PREPARE?

By taking the sample tests on the website. The only bit you can really cram for is the science paper. The rest isn't testing your knowledge so much as your analytical and logical thinking ability.

WHERE CAN I GET MORE INFO?

www.bmat.org.uk.

The 'GAMSAT'

Graduate Medical School Admissions Test

The Graduate Medical School Admissions Test was pioneered in Australia by medical schools offering graduate entry programmes. Introduced into this country in 1999, it assists in the selection for some graduate-entry programmes and is also used by Peninusula Medical School for certain applicants to its five-year course.

WHAT KIND OF TEST IS IT?

It is mostly multiple choice. It emphasises reasoning ability and critical thinking. It actively encourages students to think outside obvious parameters when seeking solutions. The ability to apply conceptual thought under time-pressure and provide the best response is at the heart of GAMSAT.

IS ANY SPECIFIC KNOWLEDGE NEEDED?

Scientific knowledge is necessary to understand the scenarios in question and the terminology. The level of knowledge is quite high. In Biology and Chemistry it is roughly equivalent to first-year degree level, whilst in Physics it is similar to A level.

WHAT QUALITIES ARE NEEDED TO SUCCEED?

Determination, flexibility of thought, scientific knowledge, the ability to write clearly and fluently are important. Analytical, logical thinking and an organised strategic approach when taking the test also help.

CAN YOU TELL ME ABOUT THE TEST?

It comes in these three sections.

- **I Reasoning in Humanities and Social Sciences**
  – 75 questions. 1 hour 40 minutes. Multiple choice questions on passages on topics evaluate critical thinking and reasoning.
- **II Written Communication** – two 30-minute essays appraise the ability to draw concepts together and express them fluently in writing.
- **III Reasoning in Biological and Physical Sciences** – 110 questions. 2 hours 50 minutes. The focus of this section is on passages and pictorial representations of data, measuring problem solving, the ability to offer hypotheses and reach reasoned conclusions.

Excellent scores in one section will not compensate for poor scores in another. Scores achieved are valid for two years.

WHICH UNIS AND COLLEGES NEED IT?

Nottingham; St George's (University of London); Peninsula Medical School; University of Wales Swansea.

WHERE CAN I GET MORE INFORMATION?

From UCAS on 01242 544730, gamsat@ucas.ac.uk or the website ucas.com. Information booklets and practice tests are available from August/September 2006.

WHEN AND WHERE DO I TAKE THE TEST?

The test takes place in early January 2007 at several locations in the UK.

The 'MSAT'

Medical School Admissions Test

WHAT IS ITS STRUCTURE?

MSAT (Medical School Admissions Test) was developed in consultation with medical schools for use in the selection of students into 4- and 5-year medicine degrees. MSAT scores are used in conjunction with academic results and performance at interview.

WHAT IS THE TEST LIKE?

It consists of three components with a total test time of three hours and is designed to complement academic achievement as evidenced by A level or undergraduate degree grades.

It is divided into these three sections.

- **Critical reasoning** – the context of the questions includes general interest, science and social science, with materials presented in a variety of text, diagrammatic, graphical and tabular formats. Some require basic mathematical skills. The emphasis is on the application of skills in reasoning and problem solving.
- **Interpersonal understanding** – focuses on working with and understanding people. It consists of scenarios, narratives and dialogues and is designed to assess the understanding of people, their behaviour and responses.

- **Written communication** – consists of a report-writing exercise and an essay requiring reasoned argument. Each task is graded using a set of specifically designed assessment criteria. Assessment focuses on the way ideas are integrated into a purposeful and relevant response to the task. Candidates are not assessed on the correctness of the ideas or attitudes.

HOW LONG IS EACH SECTION?

SECTION	NUMBER OF QUESTIONS	TIME IN MINUTES
1: Critical reasoning	45	65
2: Interpersonal understanding	45	55
3: Written communication	2	60

WHICH UNIVERSITIES AND COLLEGES USE IT?

King's College London (University of London); Queen Mary, University of London; University of Warwick.

WHERE AND WHEN DO I TAKE IT?

There are venues throughout the UK and it takes place in late November.

HOW DO I GET MORE INFORMATION?

Go to www.acer.edu.au.

The 'UKCAT'

UK Clinical Aptitude Test

The UK Clinical Aptitude Test (UKCAT) will be used in the selection process by a consortium of medical and dental schools for entry in 2007, including deferred entry for 2008. The test helps universities make more informed choices amongst the many highly qualified applicants for their medical and dentistry programmes. Its aim is to ensure candidates selected have the most appropriate abilities, attitudes and professional behaviours.

WHAT KIND OF TEST IS IT?

It is designed to test aptitude rather than simply academic achievement. It tests the mental abilities and behavioural attributes universities regard as important. It is delivered via computer, but will require minimum computer knowledge.

WHAT IS ITS STRUCTURE?

It consists of these four multiple choice subtests.

- **Verbal Reasoning** – about arriving at a reasoned conclusion over written information.
- **Quantitative Reasoning** – solving numerical problems.
- **Abstract Reasoning** – assesses the ability to use both convergent and divergent thinking.
- **Problem Solving** – assesses the ability to deal with a variety of information, infer relationships, make judgements and respond appropriately.

HOW LONG DOES IT TAKE?

Less than two hours.

HOW ABOUT REGISTRATION AND TEST DATES?

There is no fixed date for sitting the exam, but it must be before 28 September 2006. There are over 150 centres at which it can be taken across the UK. Registration is available only online at www.ukcat.ac.uk and the cost is £60 within the UK and EU and £95 for other candidates. It is recommended candidates schedule to sit the UKCAT in July and register in June 2006.

CAN I PREPARE MYSELF FOR THE TEST?

Preparation is neither necessary nor desirable. The test does not draw on any particular body of knowledge.

WHICH DENTAL SCHOOLS NEED UKCAT?

Cardiff; Dundee; Glasgow; King's College London (University of London); Manchester; Newcastle; Queen Mary, University of London; Sheffield.

WHICH MEDICAL SCHOOLS NEED UKCAT?

Aberdeen; Birmingham; Brighton and Sussex; Cardiff; Dundee; Durham; East Anglia; Edinburgh; Glasgow; Hull York; Keele; Kings College London (University of London); Leeds; Leicester; Manchester; Newcastle; Nottingham; Oxford (graduate); Peninsula (undergraduate); Queen Mary, University of London; Sheffield; Southampton; St Andrews; St George's (University of London) (undergraduate).

The interview

You may or may not be called for an interview as part of the selection process. Many institutions prefer not to interview people, as it's a very subjective and time-consuming process. However, some interview candidates as a matter of process, and others interview to clarify some aspect of a candidate's application – for example, if you're an overseas student in the UK, to check your communication skills, or if your grades are borderline.

If you are called for interview, the key areas they are likely to cover will be:

- evidence of your scientific ability
- your capacity to study hard
- your commitment to medicine or dentistry, best shown by work experience
- your awareness of current issues in the news that may have an impact on your chosen field of study, for example, the EU Working Time Directive and its effect on junior doctors' hours, the issue of access to NHS dentistry or the Modernising Medical Careers initiative
- your manual dexterity, if you're applying for dentistry.

SAMPLE INTERVIEW QUESTIONS

- How would you feel about treating a heavy smoker suffering from cancer? (To explore your approach to 'ethical' issues.)

- Can you give us some examples of your manual dexterity? (One for the dentists – good answers include playing the piano or violin, or sewing.)

- What do you think of the changes to junior doctors' working hours? (To test your awareness of what's going on in your chosen field.)

Work experience

How much does it count? Ask any medical or dental admissions tutor about the importance of work experience on a candidate's application and they'll all agree – work experience shows a real, rather than theoretical, interest in your chosen profession. An absence of work experience shows questionable commitment to your choice of career.

Work experience is especially useful to help you find out what you want to do. Since medicine (more than dentistry) is such a long course of study, it is important for you to find out early on if it could really be a career for you. Given the choice, admissions tutors prefer to see examples of long-term work experience rather than the odd week here and there.

WHAT KINDS OF SCHEMES EXIST?

Once you're on your undergraduate course, your 'rotations', ie placements in various hospital departments, will automatically give you the experience you need. As a sixth former, the good news is that more and more universities and hospitals are running short work experience schemes, from **'taster' days** to formal periods of work observation or **'shadowing' schemes** in hospitals that allow you to 'shadow' a surgeon or doctor in a particular department. Competition for the in-hospital schemes is stiff, so you'll need to apply early. You'll also have to apply directly through the hospital's medical staffing or human resources departments. 'Taster' schemes are usually offered on a first come, first served basis, and charge a fee. Ask your careers adviser to give you details of these schemes. Dental students should also try spending time at their local dental practice; for example, helping out in reception or as support for the dental nurses.

HOW CAN IT HELP YOUR PERSONAL STATEMENT?

As part of the university application process, you'll be asked to write a personal statement about yourself, setting out which subject you'd like to study, why you'd like to study it, and what skills and experience you bring that would make you a good student for the course and a great potential doctor or dentist. This is where your work experience will help you stand out.

WHAT IF YOU'VE ONLY GOT NON-MEDICAL WORK EXPERIENCE?

Don't worry – it will still be useful to include it in any applications you make. The trick is to pull out the professional and personal skills you have developed that are of relevance to the work of a doctor or dentist.

WHICH WORK EXPERIENCE?

Examples of the kinds of work experience of use to your medical/dental school application:

- shadowing a hospital doctor
- helping out in a care home
- working on reception or as support to dental nurses in a local dental practice
- working as a first-aider in Scouts
- working as a hospital auxiliary.

Cost of higher education

Please note that the figures below are correct at the time of going to press. Wherever you live in the UK, we strongly advise that you check out your own government website.

ENGLAND

The cost of going to university or college can be very difficult to calculate, as accommodation, travel, books and course fees can vary. Year-on-year living costs are on average around £6,000-£7,000, but on top of that come tuition fees. The British Medical Association advises that students in the fifth year of medical school have an average debt of £20,172 and those in the final year of a six-year course owe £22,365. But remember that as a would-be doctor or dentist, you will have studied longer and will be earning more than many other graduates. The good news is that you can receive financial help for both. Many students are entitled to help to pay for some or all of their course tuition fees, which for 2007 entry will not be paid up-front or while they are studying. Exactly how much you pay will depend on your income and that of your household and when you start your course. The figures shown below are subject to annual increases in line with inflation and will be finalised nearer the time.

From 2006, most universities and colleges of higher education will charge the maximum fee allowed by the government for home-based students, £3,000 a year, if they satisfy the criteria set down by OFFA (Office of Fair Access), for provision of bursaries for the less well-off. Some universities and colleges are planning to charge significantly less for their tuition fees.

An income-assessed non-repayable maintenance grant of up to £2,700 will be provided. Again the amount you will receive depends on your income or that of the household. If an institution sets variable course fees at the limit of £3,000 and you are entitled to the full maintenance grant, then the university or college must offer a minimum of £300 via bursaries to ensure that the cost of higher education is covered.

Your course fees are not repayable until after completion of your course, and then only once you are working with a salary over the new threshold of £15,000 a year.

The UCAS website (www.ucas.com) shows individual course fees. You will also find further information about bursaries and scholarships offered by the universities and colleges, on a course-by-course basis. Many of these are set to be very generous.

Although the cost of higher education may appear steep, don't forget about the extra financial help available from the government. It is expected that almost half of all new students will benefit from some or all of the maintenance grant. There are also non-repayable grants for those with a disability, with children or with severe hardship.

For latest information, see
www.dfes.gov.uk/studentsupport/students/index.shtml.
www.direct.gov.uk
www.offa.org.uk

For detailed fee and bursary information on each UCAS course, see www.ucas.com/search/index.html

WALES

From 2007/8, Welsh institutions will be able to charge up to £3,070 in annual deferred flexible fees.
If you normally live in Wales or the European Union (outside the UK) and choose to study in Wales, you will be entitled to a tuition fee grant of £1,845 from the Welsh Assembly Government, which does not have to be repaid. You can defer the remaining £1,225 fee contribution by taking out a loan for that amount which does not need to be repaid until after you have completed your studies and are earning at least £15,000 a year.

The new arrangements, when introduced in 2007/8, will apply to second-year students who enter higher education in 2006, as well as those starting in 2007.

For latest information, see
www.studentfinancewales.co.uk.

For detailed fee and bursary information on each UCAS course, see www.ucas.com/search/index.html.

NORTHERN IRELAND

As in England, variable tuition fees of up to £3,000 will be charged and again will be covered by a loan, payable only when you are working and earning over £15,000 a year. An income-assessed non-repayable maintenance grant will be provided, dependent on your household income and your normal place of residence. If this is Northern Ireland, the grant will be up to £3,200 per year, compared with £2,700 per year for students from England and Wales and £2,000 for students from Scotland.

As in England, each institution that charges the full £3,000 fee must provide a bursary of at least £300 to students receiving the full maintenance grant. However, as elsewhere in the UK, more generous scholarships and bursaries are being offered by universities and colleges.

For latest information, see www.delni.gov.uk/.

For detailed fee and bursary information on each UCAS course, see www.ucas.com/search/index.html.

SCOTLAND

Arrangements for students living in Scotland are different to the rest of the UK. If you live in Scotland and are starting your first full-time degree, HND, HNC or certain diploma courses in Scotland, you will not pay any course tuition fees and you may be eligible for a non-repayable bursary of up to £2,455 a year, depending on your household income. You can also apply for a partly means-tested loan to help with living costs. If you are a lone parent or have dependants, you may be able to get an extra, non-repayable grant.

Around half of all full-time students will pay a 'graduate endowment' once they have finished their courses; the figure for students who started in 2005 was £2,216. These amounts will increase by the rate of inflation for students starting in future years.

EU (outside the UK) students who choose to study in Scotland will have the same arrangements as those living in Scotland.

Scottish Students who study elsewhere in the UK

Scottish students who choose to study elsewhere in the UK are liable for an income-assessed contribution to the fees charged by individual universities and colleges. Universities and colleges in England, Wales and Northern Ireland may charge fees of up to £3,000 per year. There is a bursary for Scottish students who study elsewhere in the UK. It is currently worth up to £2,000, depending on family circumstances. Students can apply for a non-means-tested fee loan to cover the cost of tuition fees.

Students from elsewhere in the UK studying in Scotland

Students from other parts of the UK who study in Scotland will be liable to pay tuition fees of £1,700 a year (£2,700 for Medicine). The Scottish Executive will offer a partial fee waiver to students from low-income families.

Further information is available on the Scottish Executive's website at www.scotland.gov.uk.

This is only a brief description of the arrangements in Scotland. Full information is available from the Student Awards Agency for Scotland (SAAS) on its website – www.saas.gov.uk – or telephone 0845 1111711 or email saas.geu@scotland.gsi.gov.uk.

For detailed fee and bursary information on each UCAS course, see www.ucas.com/search/index.html

International students

Applications to medical and dental schools in the UK are made via the UCAS website. UCAS accepts applications from all students, irrespective of their country of origin, for a set fee of £5 for one application or £15 for up to six choices (with a maximum of four choices in medicine or dentistry).

Before you apply, you should contact individual medical/dental schools in the UK, to find out if your qualifications meet their current entrance requirements. For more information on equivalent and acceptable qualifications email quals@ucas.ac.uk or phone +44 (0) 1242 544900.

All nationals wishing to come to the UK for more than six months must get 'entry clearance' **before** they come. In general, overseas students coming to take an undergraduate degree that lasts one academic year or longer, and finishes in the summer are given a visa until the 31 October following the summer in which their course ends. For more information see the UK's Immigration and Nationality Directorate www.ind.homeoffice.gov.uk or www.ukvisas.gov.uk.

WHAT LEVEL OF ENGLISH?

To study medicine or dentistry in the UK, you will have to have a high level of English – typically IELTS 6+. Each individual medical/dental school sets its own entry requirement in English, so please check with them before applying. UCAS provides a list of English language qualifications and grades that are acceptable to most UK universities. Go to www.ucas.com/student/index.html and click on 'international students'.

If you already have a degree from your own country, and want to train as a doctor in the UK, you will also have to take **PLAB** (Professional and Linguistic Assessment Board) exams, which are similar to the exams taken by final year UK medical school students. NB: while there are shortages of consultants and GPs in the UK, there are generally fewer shortages in the training grades. This means that there is stiff competition among UK graduates for clinical attachments in hospitals, so overseas doctors may find them difficult to secure, and some NHS trusts also expect overseas doctors to pay for them. Most British Council offices will have information and advice about entry to UK medical and dental schools.

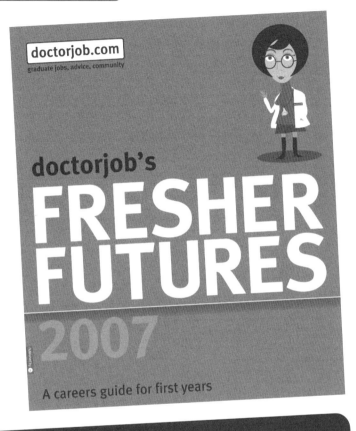
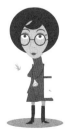

www.ucas.com

helping you into higher education

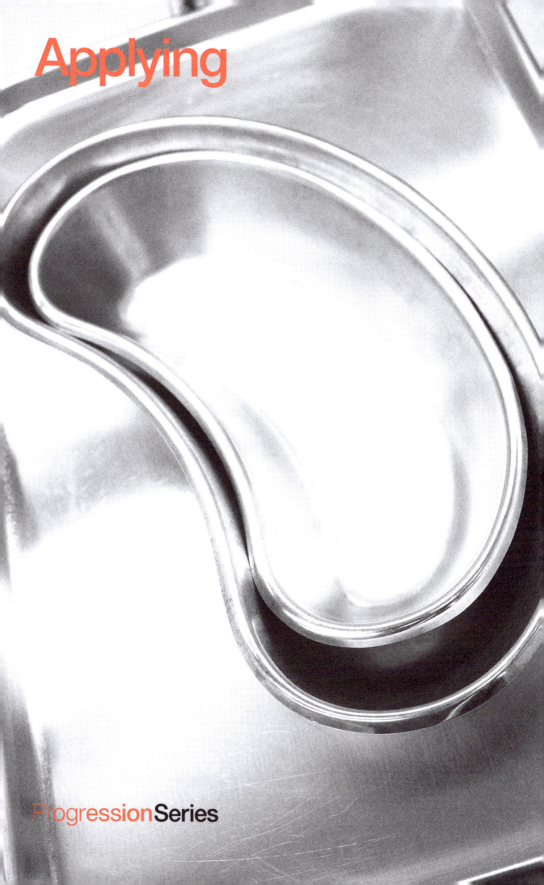

Applying

How to apply via UCAS

You can apply to up to **six** institutions or courses for your undergraduate degree (with a maximum of four choices in medicine or dentistry). If you're applying through your school or sixth-form college, you should apply online at ucas.com via Apply – a secure, online application system that is:

- easy to access – all you need is an internet connection
- easy to use – you don't have to complete your application all in one go: you can save the sections as you complete them and come back to it later
- easy to monitor – once you've applied through Apply, you can use Track to check the progress of your application, including any decisions from universities or colleges, and you can make your replies online.

You can only submit one UCAS application in each year's application cycle.

The following diagram is a step-by-step guide to introduce you to the application process:

APPLYING VIA YOUR SCHOOL OR COLLEGE

1 GET SCHOOL OR COLLEGE 'BUZZWORD'

Ask your UCAS application co-ordinator (may be your sixth form tutor) for your school or college UCAS 'buzzword'. This is a password for the school or college.

2 REGISTER

Log on to www.ucas.com/apply and click on **Student login**. Click on register. The form will automatically generate a username for you, but you'll have to come with a password and security question and answer.

3 COMPLETE FIVE SECTIONS

Complete the sections of the application. To access any section, click on the section name at the top of the screen and follow the instructions. The sections are:

Courses – ie which courses you'd like to apply for

Education – ie your education to date

Employment – for example, work experience, holiday jobs

About you – some more personal details about you

Personal statement – see below.

4 PASS TO REFEREE

Once you've completed all the sections, send your application electronically to your referee (normally your form tutor). They'll check it, approve it and add their reference to it, and will then send it to UCAS on your behalf.

5 APPLY BY

- 15 October for medicine, dentistry, Oxford and Cambridge courses
- Mid January for all other courses.

NOT APPLYING VIA A SCHOOL OR COLLEGE

For example, you're a mature or overseas student – you can follow the same steps, but, as you can't supply a 'buzzword', you'll just be asked a few extra questions to check you are eligible to apply and you'll have to supply a reference from someone who knows you well enough to state that you're suitable for higher education.

Making your application

We want this to run smoothly for you and we also want to process your application as quickly as possible. You can help us to do this by remembering to do the following.

- Check the on-time dates for applications – see below and the applications flowchart on page 108.
- Allow plenty of time for completing your application – including enough time for your referee to complete the reference section.
- Help text will guide you through the process.
- Consider what each question is actually asking for.
- Ask a teacher, parent, friend or careers adviser to review your application before you submit it – particularly the personal statement.
- Pay special attention to questions that ask you about your interests and experience.

- If you have extra information that will not fit on your application, send it direct to your chosen universities or colleges after we have sent you your welcome letter with your personal identifier and application number.
- Print and keep a copy of the final version of your application, in case you are asked questions on it at an interview.

WHEN TO APPLY

Make a note of these important dates for your diary.

- **1 September 2006**

  Opening date for receiving applications

- **15 October 2006**

  On-time date for applications to medicine and dentistry courses, Oxford University and the University of Cambridge

- **15 January 2007**

  Closing date for on-time applications, but not applications from outside the UK or EU.

- **30 June 2007**

  Last date that we must receive all other applications, including those from outside the UK or EU before Clearing

YOUR APPLICATION

Applications through UCAS are made online using Apply on our website www.ucas.com. Apply is a secure, web-based application system, which has been designed for all our applicants whether they are applying through a school, college, Careers Scotland, Connexions or British Council office registered with us. Applicants in the UK and elsewhere in the world who are not applying through one of these organisations can also use Apply.

- You can use Apply anywhere that has access to the internet.
- Important details like date of birth and course codes will be checked by Apply. It will alert you if they are not valid.
- The text for your personal statement and reference can be copied and pasted into your application.
- You can change your application at any time before it is completed and sent to UCAS.
- You can print and preview your application at any time.

- Your school, college, Connexions or Careers Scotland office can choose different payment methods. For example, they may want us to bill them, or you may be able to pay online by debit or credit card.

Deferred entry

If you want to apply for deferred entry in 2008, perhaps because you want to take a year out between school or college and higher education, you should check that the university or college will accept a deferred entry application. Occasionally, tutors are not happy to accept students who take a gap year, because it interrupts the flow of their learning. If you apply, you must meet the conditions of any offers by 31 August 2007. If you accept a place for 2008 entry and then change your mind, you cannot reapply through us in the 2008 entry cycle, unless you withdraw your original application by 30 September 2007.

Invisibility of choices

Universities and colleges cannot see details of the other choices on your application until you reply to any offers or you have not been successful at any of your choices.

You can only submit one UCAS application in each year's application cycle.

The personal statement

Next to choosing your courses, this section of your application will take up most of your time. It is of immense importance as many colleges and universities rely solely on the information in the UCAS application, rather than interviews and admissions tests, when selecting students. The personal statement can be the deciding factor in whether or not they offer you a place. If it is an institution that interviews, it could be the deciding factor in whether you get called for interview. And keep a copy of your personal statement – if you are called for interview, you will almost certainly be asked questions based on it.

Tutors will look carefully at your exam results, actual and predicted, your referee's statement and your own personal statement. Remember, they are looking for reasons to offer you a place – try to give them every opportunity to do so! Remember, applying on time is vital.

A SALES DOCUMENT

The personal statement is your opportunity to sell yourself, so do so. The university or college admissions tutor who reads your personal statement wants to get a rounded picture of you to decide whether you will make an interesting member of the university or college both academically and socially. They want to know more about you than the subjects you are studying at school.

HOW TO IMPRESS

Don't be put off by the blank space. The secret is to cover key areas that admissions tutors always look for. Include things like hobbies and work experience, especially if they are linked in some way to the type of course you are applying for. You could talk about your career plans and interesting things you might have done outside the classroom. Have you belonged to sports teams, orchestras or held positions of responsibility? Maybe you've been a school play stalwart or done loads of community service. If you are a mature student, talk about the work you have done and the skills you have gathered or how you have juggled bringing up a family – that is evidence of time management skills. Whoever you are, make sure you explain what appeals to you about the course you are applying for. The medicine and dentistry profiles in this book will also provide you with some idea of what qualities universities and colleges are looking for.

REMEMBER

Those applying for medicine and dentistry are going into areas with more applicants than places. Your first step is to prompt the admissions tutor who reads your application to offer you an interview, so it is important to gear your statement to your intended area of study (because other people will) and to treat your experience as valuable and positive. Even those institutions that do not interview everyone to whom they intend to offer places look very closely at this section of the application. They want to know what you have gained from your experiences, what you have achieved and hope to achieve. They will be looking to put ticks against your name, so don't waste your time providing them with reasons to put crosses.

| WHAT THEY LOOK FOR... | WHAT TO TELL THEM... |

- Your reasons for wanting to take this course
- Your communication skills – how you express yourself in the personal statement
- Relevant experience – ie experience that's related to your choice of course
- Evidence of your interest in this field
- Evidence of your teamwork
- Evidence of your skills, for example, IT skills, people skills, debating and public speaking
- Other activities that show your dedication and ability to apply yourself

- why you want to do this subject
- what experience you already have in this field – for example work experience, school projects, hobbies, voluntary work
- the skills and qualities you have as a person that would make you a good student, for example, anything that shows your dedication, communication ability, academic achievement, initiative
- anything that shows you can knuckle down and apply yourself, for example running a marathon, raising money for charity
- if you're taking a gap year, why and, if possible, what you're going to do during it
- about your other interests and activities away from studying – to show you're a 'rounded' person

Extra

Extra allows you to make additional choices, one at a time. It is completely optional, and is designed to encourage you to continue researching and choosing courses if you need to. The courses available through Extra will be highlighted on Course Search, www.ucas.com. Or you can contact universities and colleges to ask them directly.

WHO IS ELIGIBLE?

You will be eligible for Extra if:

- you have had unsuccessful or withdrawal decisions from all six of your choices
- you have cancelled your outstanding choices and hold no offers
- you have received decisions from all six choices and have declined all offers made to you.

If, as an applicant for medicine or dentistry, you have used only four of the six possible UCAS choices, you can add two further choices (not in your original subject area). Only after using all six choices will you become eligible for Extra.

It is comparatively rare for institutions to advertise vacancies in medicine and dentistry in Extra, but if you do find a vacancy for which you wish to apply and have been unsuccessful in all your original choices, ring the UCAS Customer Service Unit on 0870 1122211 for advice. They will be able to help you.

How does it work?

We write to you and explain what to do if you are eligible for Extra. If you are eligible, you should:

- see a special Extra button on your Track screen
- check on Course Search for courses that are available through Extra
- choose one that you would like to apply for and enter the details on your Track screen.

When you have finished, a copy of your application will be sent to the university or college.

What happens next?

We give universities and colleges 21 days to consider your Extra application. During this time, you cannot be considered by another university or college. After 21 days you can refer yourself to a different university or college if you wish, but it is a good idea to ring the one currently considering you before doing so. If you are made an offer, you can choose whether or not to accept it. If you are currently studying for examinations, any offer that you receive is likely to be an offer conditional on exam grades.

If you decide to accept a conditional offer, you will not be able to take any further part in Extra.

If you already have your examination results, it is possible that a university or college may make an unconditional offer.

If you accept an unconditional offer, you will be placed.

If you decide to decline the offer or the university or college decides it cannot make you an offer, you will be given another opportunity to use Extra, time permitting.

Your Extra button will be reactivated on Track.

Once you have accepted an offer in Extra, you are committed to it in the same way as you would be with an offer through the main UCAS system. Conditional offers made through Extra will be treated in the same way as other conditional offers, when your examination results become available.

If your results do not meet the conditions and the university or college decides that they cannot confirm your Extra offer, you will automatically become eligible for Clearing.

If you are unsuccessful, decline an offer, or do not receive an offer, or 21 days has elapsed since choosing a course through Extra, you can make a further application.

From 1 October – 30 June

Applicants informed as they become eligible for Extra.

From mid-March – 7 July

The Extra service is available to eligible applicants via Track at www.ucas.com.

The tariff

BACKGROUND

The UCAS Tariff is a points score system for qualifications for entry to higher education. The object of the tariff is to:

- report your achievement for entry to higher education by giving numerical values to qualifications
- establish equivalence between different types of qualifications
- provide comparisons between applicants with different types of achievement.

The development of the tariff has provided the opportunity for an inclusive points system that recognises a wide range of qualifications, including elements like music grades.

HOW DO I SCORE TARIFF POINTS?

Briefly, you get 120 points for grade A in a six-unit qualification such as GCE A level. For this qualification, the points scores go down in steps of 20 points per grade, for example, B = 100 points, C = 80. Three-unit qualifications such as GCE AS, have points that are half of those for six-unit qualifications, so an A grade at AS is worth 60 points, a B, 50 points and so on.

WHAT QUALIFICATIONS ARE COVERED BY THE TARIFF?

The tariff is continually developing and expanding, but at present, it includes the following qualifications for 2007 entry to higher education.

- GCE Double Award, GCE A level, GCE AS Double Award and GCE AS
- AVCE (six units), ASVCE (three units) and AVCE Double Award (12 units)
- The key skills of Application of Number, Communication and Information Technology at levels 2, 3 and 4
- The three wider key skills of Improving Own Learning and Performance, Problem Solving and Working with Others
- Free-standing Mathematics Qualifications at level 3
- Intermediate 2 and Standard Grade Credit (Scotland)
- Highers and Advanced Highers (Scotland)
- Core skills of Communication, IT, Numeracy, Problem Solving and Working with Others (Scotland)
- CACHE Diploma in Child Care and Education
- ABRSM, Guildhall, LCMM, Rockschool and Trinity Guildhall music examinations, grades 6, 7 and 8
- Institute of Financial Services, Certificate in Financial Studies (CeFS)
- BTEC National Award (six units), Certificate (12-units) and Diploma (18 units)
- Irish Leaving Certificate (ILC)
- Diploma in Foundation Studies (Art and Design)
- Welsh Baccalaureate
- Advanced Extension Awards
- OCR National Certificate (six units), Diploma (12 units) and Extended Diploma (18 units)
- BTEC Nationals in Early Years Professional Placement
- ASDAN Certificate of Personal Effectiveness (COPE)

HOW DOES THE TARIFF WORK?

The following are some of the most important principles.

- Points can be added together for any combination of qualifications, for example, a student might take a mix of GCE A level, GCE AS and AVCE qualifications, supplemented by key skills.
- Points for GCE AS are incorporated into the scores for GCE A level in the same subject.
- Points for Scottish Highers are incorporated into scores for Advanced Higher in the same subject.

- Points for key skills achievement at a lower level, for example, level 2, are incorporated into the highest level of achievement in that skill, for example, level 3 or 4, according to the circumstances.
- All certificated key skills achievement in Application of Number, Communication and IT attract points scores shown in the chart on page 105.
- Points for Scottish core skills for Intermediate 2 are incorporated into the scores for Higher core skills.

- The tariff does not cover former or legacy qualifications, including GCE A levels started before September 2002. The latter are dealt with by higher education institutions individually on the basis of grades, and not on the old discontinued points system.

HOW WIDELY IS THE TARIFF USED?

Almost three-quarters of universities and colleges in the UCAS scheme use the tariff to express their entry requirements for some or all of their courses, but because it is not compulsory for universities and colleges to use the tariff, some have chosen to express their entry requirements in terms of exam grades.

Where entry requirements are expressed in points, it may be necessary for the applicant to complete at least two six-unit qualifications or equivalent, such as two GCE A levels or a Double Award AVCE. **In other cases**, a course may ask for a certain level of pass in a specified subject, such as GCE A level chemistry at grade A, as a reflection of the importance of that subject for study of the course concerned. There are other ways in which points score entry requirements may be restricted, and you should read the information provided by individual universities or colleges carefully to check you will be fully qualified for entry.

HOW IS THE TARIFF USED?

Conditional points offers have greater flexibility than offers based on grades. This is because they give the applicant the opportunity of fulfilling the offer in a variety of ways. But you should know that universities and colleges often want to make sure applicants have the right depth of knowledge for a course. They won't let you in with points based just on qualifications at, for example, GCE AS and ASVCE. That's why they might specify in offers that applicants must have two GCE A levels, or their equivalent. In some cases, the points

from a particular qualification might not be taken into account for entry to a particular course, perhaps because the qualification is not considered relevant to that course. To recap, points offers will often require some or all of the following.

- Specified number of passes in six-unit qualifications, for example, GCE A level and AVCE.
- Achievement in a named subject, for example, GCE A level chemistry.
- Specified grade or points in one or more qualifications.

Also:

- a points offer might exclude specific qualifications
- points from key skills qualifications can be counted, unless specifically excluded by a university or college.

Remember, it is not compulsory for universities and colleges to use tariff points to make an offer of a place, and some have chosen to use points for some courses, but not for others. Indeed, there is no reason why a grade offer could not be made to one applicant and a points offer to another for the same course, if that serves the interests of clarity in each case.

Here are some examples of tariff points scores.

EXAMPLE 1		

Polly is taking three GCE A levels plus one AS qualification

GCE A level

English grade B*	100	
History grade C*	80	
Economics grade D*	60	240
*incorporating AS in each case		

GCE AS

Psychology grade B	50	50
		290

Here are some examples of tariff points score offers made by universities and colleges.

EXAMPLE 2

Richard is taking AVCE Double Award, GCE AS and key skills

AVCE Double Award

Business grade AB	220

GCE AS

French D	30

Key skills

Application of Number level 2	10	
IT level 3	20	30
Total points		**280**

EXAMPLE 3

Cara is taking four Scottish Highers, two Advanced Highers and five core skills

Scottish Highers

Mathematics C	48	
Chemistry B	60	
Physics C	48	
Geography B (incorporated in Advanced Higher)	=	**156**

Advanced Highers

Geography B (incorporating Higher)	100	
Economics B	100	200

Core skills

Five core skills (Higher)	100	100
		456

EXAMPLE 1

Maddy is taking three GCE A levels, one GCE AS and key skills.

Her offer is subject to her obtaining

A minimum of 300 UCAS tariff points including

Grade B in GCE A level Mathematics

Grade B in one further GCE A level subject

As it doesn't say that Maddy can't use key skill points, she can count them towards the offer.

EXAMPLE 2

Emma is taking AVCE Double Award, GCE AS and key skills.

Her offer is subject to her obtaining

A minimum of 220 UCAS tariff points including

Grade CC in

AVCE Double Award Information and Communications Technology

EXAMPLE 3

Ben is taking Scottish Highers and Advanced Highers.

His offer is subject to him obtaining

A minimum of 300 UCAS Tariff points including

Grade C in

Scottish Qualifications Authority Advanced Higher Italian

WHAT ELSE IS THE TARIFF USED FOR?

- By universities and colleges to compile statistical returns for the Higher Education Funding Council for England and the Higher Education Statistics Agency.
- By employers, mainly as an initial filter in the selection of applicants for graduate jobs.
- By professional bodies.

FURTHER INFORMATION

The tariff continues to be developed to include other qualifications. Updated information on the tariff can be found at www.ucas.com.
All enquiries about the tariff should be made to the UCAS Outreach department.
Tel: +44 (0)1242 544900
Fax: +44 (0)1242 544954
Email: quals@ucas.ac.uk

THE TARIFF

GCE AS/AS VCE	GCE AS Double Award	GCE A level/AVCE	GCE/AVCE Double Award	BTEC Award	BTEC Certificate	BTEC Diploma	OCR Certificate	OCR Diploma	OCR Extended Diploma	Points	Irish Higher	Irish Ordinary	Scottish Advanced Higher	Scottish Higher	Scottish Intermediate 2	Scottish Standard Grade
						DDD				360						
						DDM			D1	320						
				DD	DMM			D2/M1		280						
			AA			MMM			M2	240						
			AB						M3	220						
			BB		DM	MMP		D	P1	200						
			BC		MM	MPP		M1		180						
			CC	D	MP	PPP		M2/P1	P2	160						
			CD	M	PP			P2	P3	140						
	AA	A	DD	P						120			A			
	AB									110						
	BB	B	DE					P3		100			B			
	BC									90	A1					
	CC	C	EE				D			80			C			
										77	A2					
										72				A		
										71	B1					
	CD									70						
										64	B2					
A	DD	D					M			60				B		
										58	B3					
										52	C1					
B	DE									50						
							P			48				C		
										45	C2					
										42					A	
C	EE	E								40						
										39	C3	A1				
										38						Band 1
										35					B	
										33	D1					
D										30						Band 2
										28					C	
										26	D2	A2				
E										20	D3	B1				
										14		B2				
										7		B3				

1 The points shown are for the newly specified BTEC National Award, Certificate and Diploma introduced into centres from September 2002

2 The points for the OCR Nationals come into effect for entry to higher education in 2007 onwards

3 The points shown for the Irish Leaving Certificate, Higher and Ordinary levels, come into effect for entry to higher education in 2006 onwards

BTEC Nationals in Early Years[4]			CACHE Diploma in Child Care & Education		Diploma in Foundation Studies (Art and Design)[5]	Points	Music Examinations[6]					
Theory		Practical	Theory	Practical			Practical			Theory		
Certificate	Diploma						Grade 6	Grade 7	Grade 8	Grade 6	Grade 7	Grade 8
	DDD					320						
					Distinction	285						
	DDM					280						
	DMM		AA			240						
					Merit	225						
	MMM					220						
DD			BB			200						
					Pass	165						
DM	MMP		CC			160						
MM	MPP	D	DD	A		120						
				B		100						
MP	PPP	M	EE	C		80						
						75			D			
						70			M			
			D			60		D				
						55		M	P			
						45	D					
PP		P		E		40	M	P				
						30						D
						25	P					M
						20					D	P
						15				D	M	
						10				M	P	
						5				P		

4   The new allocation of points for the theory and practical elements of the BTEC Nationals in Early Years comes into effect for entry to higher education in **2007** onwards

5   Points for the Diploma in Foundation Studies (Art and Design) come into effect for entry to higher education in **2006** onwards

6   Points shown are for ABRSM, Guildhall, LCMM, Rockschool and Trinity Guildhall advanced level music examinations

Free-standing Maths[7]	IFS CeFS[8]	ASDAN COPE[9]	Advanced Extension Awards[10]	Points	Core Skills[11]	Key Skills[12]	Welsh Baccalaureate Core[13]
				120			Pass
		Pass		70			
	A			60			
	B			50			
	C		Distinction	40			
	D			30		Level 4	
A	E		Merit	20	Higher	Level 3	
B				17			
C				13			
D				10	Int 2	Level 2	
E				7			

7   Covers free-standing Mathematics qualifications – Additional Maths, Using and Applying Statistics, Working with Algebraic and Graphical Techniques, Modelling with Calculus

8   Points shown are for the revised Institute of Financial Services Certificate in Financial Studies (CeFS) taught from September 2003

9   Points for ASDAN's Certificate of Personal Effectiveness (COPE) come into effect for entry to higher education in **2007**

10   Points for Advanced Extension Awards are over and above those gained from the A level grade and come into effect for entry to higher education in **2006**

11   Covers the five Scottish Core Skills – Communication, Information Technology, Numeracy, Problem Solving and Working with Others

12   Covers the three main Key Skills subjects – Application of Number, Communication and Information Technology with the three Wider Key Skills (Improving Own Learning and Performance, Problem Solving, Working With Others) coming into effect for **2007** entry

13   Points for the Core are awarded only when a candidate achieves the Welsh Baccalaureate Advanced Diploma

Contacts and useful information

USEFUL CONTACTS

- For information relating to the UCAS application process, please contact UCAS Customer Services on 0870 1122211.

Careers advice

- Connexions is for you if you live in England, are aged 13-19 and want advice on getting to where you want to be in life.

  Connexions personal advisers can give you information, advice and practical help with all sorts of things, like choosing subjects at school or mapping out your future career options. They can help you with anything that might be affecting you at school, college, work or in your personal or family life. For where to find your local office, look at www.connexions.gov.uk.

- learndirect
  Not sure what job you want? Need help to decide which course to do? Give learndirect a call on 0800 100 900 or, for Scotland, 0800 100 9000.
  www.learndirect.co.uk
  www.learndirectscotland.com

- Careers Scotland provides a starting point for anyone looking for careers information, advice or guidance.
  www.careers-scotland.org.uk

- Careers Wales
  Wales' national all-age careers guidance service.
  www.careerswales.com

- Northern Ireland Careers Service website for the new, all-age careers guidance service in Northern Ireland.
  www.careersserviceni.com

YEAR OUT

▪ For useful information on taking a year out, see www.gapyear.com.

The Year Out Group website is packed with information and guidance for young people and their parents and advisers.
www.yearoutgroup.org

STUDENT SUPPORT

▪ DfES (Department for Education and Skills) in England and Wales.
Further information is available in *Financial Support for Higher Education Students in 2006/07.*
To obtain a copy, contact your Local Education Authority (LEA) or the DfES Information Line on 0800 731 9133. You can also download it from the website.
www.dfes.gov.uk/studentsupport/

Information for Scotland and Northern Ireland is given below.

▪ The Student Loans Company
Provides essential information on student loans.
www.slc.co.uk

▪ Local Education Authority (LEA)
For a list of LEA addresses in England:
www.dfes.gov.uk/leas/.

▪ Student Awards Agency for Scotland (SAAS)
Find out more about fees and loans from the booklet *Student Support in Scotland.* You can obtain one by calling 0845 1111711 or by writing to SAAS, Gyleview House, 3 Redheughs Rigg, South Gyle, Edinburgh EH12 9HH.
www.saas.gov.uk

▪ Department for Employment and Learning (DEL)
If you live in Northern Ireland, your Education and Library Board will assess you. For more information, you can download a booklet *Financial Support for Higher Education Students,* published by DEL.
www.delni.gov.uk

APPLICATIONS FOR UCAS COURSES

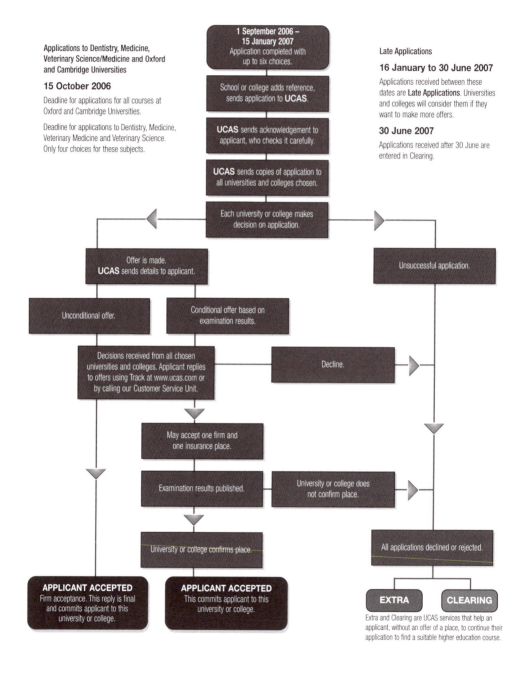

Applications to Dentistry, Medicine, Veterinary Science/Medicine and Oxford and Cambridge Universities

15 October 2006

Deadline for applications for all courses at Oxford and Cambridge Universities.

Deadline for applications to Dentistry, Medicine, Veterinary Medicine and Veterinary Science. Only four choices for these subjects.

1 September 2006 – 15 January 2007
Application completed with up to six choices.

School or college adds reference, sends application to **UCAS**.

UCAS sends acknowledgement to applicant, who checks it carefully.

UCAS sends copies of application to all universities and colleges chosen.

Each university or college makes decision on application.

Offer is made.
UCAS sends details to applicant.

Unconditional offer.

Conditional offer based on examination results.

Decisions received from all chosen universities and colleges. Applicant replies to offers using Track at www.ucas.com or by calling our Customer Service Unit.

Decline.

May accept one firm and one insurance place.

Examination results published.

University or college does not confirm place.

University or college confirms place.

Unsuccessful application.

All applications declined or rejected.

APPLICANT ACCEPTED
Firm acceptance. This reply is final and commits applicant to this university or college.

APPLICANT ACCEPTED
This commits applicant to this university or college.

EXTRA   **CLEARING**

Extra and Clearing are UCAS services that help an applicant, without an offer of a place, to continue their application to find a suitable higher education course.

Late Applications

16 January to 30 June 2007

Applications received between these dates are **Late Applications**. Universities and colleges will consider them if they want to make more offers.

30 June 2007

Applications received after 30 June are entered in Clearing.

Useful publications

We have a range of publications that can help throughout the application process, and we have identified a number of other publications that we feel can supply applicants, parents and advisers with the information they require to find places in higher education.

The publications listed below are available through UCAS Media Publication Services unless otherwise stated. (Postage and packing charges are not included in the price. When placing an order with the UCAS Media Publication Services team, you will be advised of the postage and packing charge.)

UCAS Media

Tel: +44 (0)1242 544610

Fax: +44 (0)1242 544806

Email: publicationservices@ucas.ac.uk

Website: www.ucasbooks.com

Post: UCAS Media
Publication Services team
PO Box 130
Cheltenham
Gloucestershire
GL52 3ZF

NEED HELP COMPLETING YOUR APPLICATION?

How to Complete your UCAS Application 2007 Entry

A must for anyone applying through UCAS. Contains advice on the preparation needed, a step-by-step guide to filling out the UCAS application, information on the UCAS process and useful tips for completing the personal statement.
Published by Trotman
Price £11.99

CHOOSING COURSES

'Progression to...' guides 2007 entry

UCAS, in conjunction with GTI Specialist Publishers, has produced four other new titles as well as Medicine and Dentistry to help you access good quality, useful information on some of the most competitive subject areas. The books cover advice on applying through UCAS, routes to qualifications, course details, job prospects, case studies and career advice. Published by UCAS.

Progression to Art and Design
Progression to Economics, Finance and Accountancy
Progression to Engineering and Mathematics
Progression to Law
Complete Progression set (five titles) £59.99
All Guides £14.99

UCAS Directory 2007 entry

Contains all the course data you need to complete the UCAS application.
Price £10 for individual copies of the printed version

Scottish Guide 2007

The directory for higher education in Scotland. Lists the courses available and contains information about the institutions offering them and their likely offers.
Published by UCAS
Price £14.95

UCAS Parent Guide

Available through Customer Services – call 0870 1122211.

Getting in, Getting on 2007 entry

Conventions have become a central part of the post-16 careers education and guidance programme. This publication has been designed to be used before, during and after the event. It can make a difference.
Published by UCAS
Price £15

Open Days 2006

Attending open days, taster courses and higher education conventions is an important part of the application process. This publication makes planning attendance at these events quick and easy.
Published annually by UCAS in association with Cambridge Occupational Analysts
Price £3

How to Get into Social Work 2007

A guide to help you make your application in social work. Produced in association with the Care Council for Wales (CCW), the General Social Care Council (GSCC), the Northern Ireland Social Care Council (NISCC) and the Scottish Social Services Council (SSSC).
Price £9.95

Initial Teacher Training 2007

An essential research tool for potential teachers. Contains details of undergraduate and postgraduate teacher training programmes offered in England, Wales and Scotland. Produced in association with the Training and Development Agency for Schools (TDA), the Higher Education Funding Council for Wales (HEFCW) and the Scottish Executive Education Department (SEED).
Price £9.99

Getting into Guides

Clear and concise guides to help applicants secure places in chosen areas. Includes qualifications required, advice on applying, tests, interviews and case studies. Gives an honest view on each subject and institution, and discusses current issues and careers.

- Getting into Business & Management
- Getting into Oxford & Cambridge
- Getting into Physiotherapy Courses
- Getting into Psychology Courses
- Getting into Veterinary School

Published by Trotman
Price £11.99

DEFERRING ENTRY

A Year Off... A Year On?

Essential for anyone considering time out from education. Packed with ideas on what to do, where to go and how to use your time constructively.
Published by Lifetime Careers and UCAS
Price £10.99

CHOOSING WHERE TO STUDY

The Virgin Alternative Guide to British Universities 2007

An insider's guide to choosing a university or college. Written by students and using independent statistics, this guide evaluates what you get from a higher education institution.
Published by Virgin
Price £15.99

Disabled Students' Guide to University

Details academic and cultural provision at each university for disabled students, plus information on facilities and the local area. Also includes case studies and contact details for universities and colleges.
Published by Trotman
Price £21.99

The Student Book 2007

Contains the answers to questions that prospective students have. Including the best and worst features of an institution, hotspots for student nightlife, finance and debt advice, case studies of current students and employment and drop-out rates.
Published by Trotman
Price £16.99

Student Life: A Survival Guide

The guide for anyone beginning, or soon to begin, a course at university or college.
Published by Lifetime Careers and UCAS
Price £10.99

The Times Good University Guide 2007

An authoritative guide to all the crucial facts and figures to help students find the best university and college for the subject they want to study. Includes advice and information on bursaries and scholarships, student finance and graduate prospects. Also includes university and college profiles, league tables and information specifically designed for international students.
Published by HarperCollins
Price £15.99

The Push Guide to Which University 2007

Independent, objective and incisive. Written by students and recent graduates to provide an honest view of university. With facts and figures, as well as how to make the right choice and how to apply.
Published by Nelson Thornes
Price £15.99

The Push Guide to Choosing a University

A pocket-sized guide that explains all the differences between higher education institutions and how they affect life as a student. It's also packed with tips on choosing a course, the application process and student funding. Perhaps best of all, it has Push's unique Choose your Top University questionnaire (which can be used with Push Online's unique shortlisting software) to help design your ideal institution and to match you up with those that come closest to your requirements.
3rd edition.
Published by Hodder Arnold
Price £4.99

FINANCIAL INFORMATION

The Student Finance Guide

This book offers guidance and advice for students, aspiring students and parents, on a range of subjects, including top-up fees, living costs, grants, subsidies and bursaries, working through university and college and paying off debts. Published by Kogan Page. Price £9.99

Undergraduate Courses and Funding Guide 2007

Contains all you need to know about awards, bursaries and scholarships for undergraduate and postgraduate students.
Price £3.95

Students' Money Matters 2006

With graduate debt increasing, this guide provides invaluable information for students about loans, overdrafts, work experience, jobs and accommodation. Also includes advice on budgeting, borrowing and the new top-up fees.
Published by Trotman
Price £14.99

CAREERS PLANNING

What Do Graduates Do? 2006

A comprehensive look at the graduate employment market. Providing data detailing the first destinations of first-degree and HND graduates, this guide profiles how many leavers enter employment or further study and how many are unemployed. To complement the data, there are articles and editorial for each subject area.
Published by Graduate Prospects
Price £14.95

'Careers with' guides

These comprehensive guides look at the wide range of opportunities open to graduates. They are designed to help students of all ages make the right choices about their education and careers.
▪ Careers with a Science Degree
▪ Careers with an Arts or Humanities Degree
Published by Lifetime Careers
Price £10.99

Please note that all publications incur a postage and packing charge. All information was correct at the time of printing.

TARGET
Medicine 2007

Find out more about a career in medicine

TARGET *Medicine* has all the information you need to know about life as a doctor. It includes inspirational profiles of doctors at all stages of their careers and information about the different specialty areas you can go into, from paediatrics to surgery.

Pick up your FREE copy from November 2006 at your university careers service or order a copy online at **doctorjob.com/products**. Don't forget to visit **doctorjob.com/medicine**. It's packed with information about what it's like to work as a doctor.

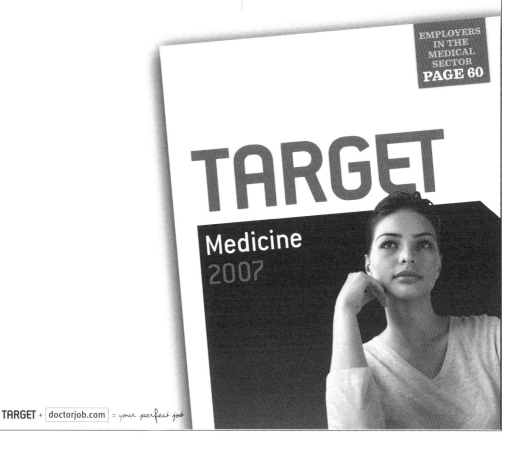

EMPLOYERS IN THE MEDICAL SECTOR
PAGE 60

TARGET

Medicine
2007

TARGET + doctorjob.com = *your perfect job*

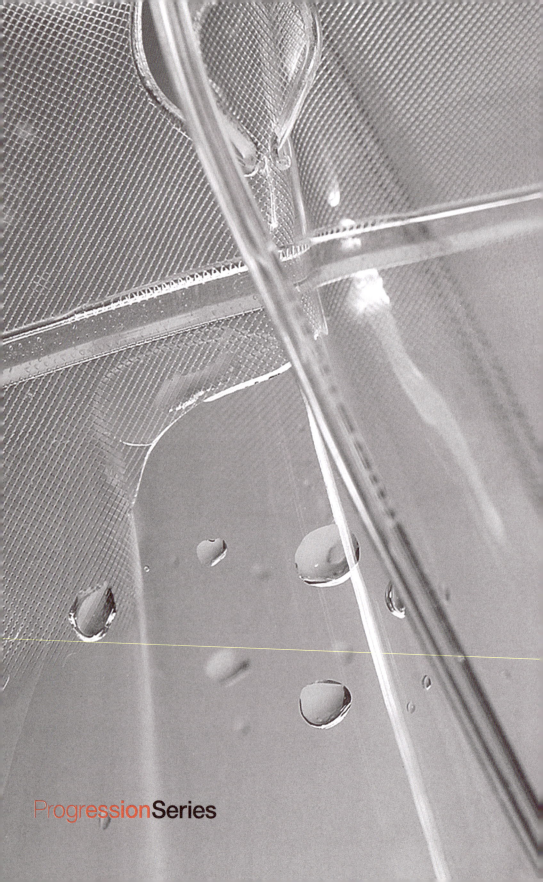

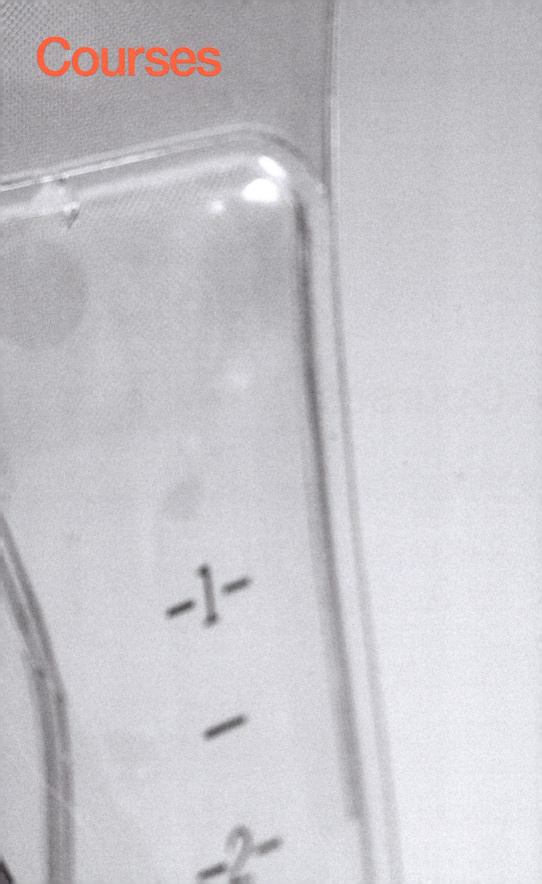

Courses

Courses

Keen to get started on your medicine or dentistry career? This section contains details of the various degree courses available at UK institutions.

EXPLAINING THE LIST OF COURSES

We list the universities and colleges by their UCAS institution codes. If there is a section for non-UCAS entries, colleges are listed alphabetically. Within each institution, courses are listed first by award type (such as BA, BSc, FdA, HND, MA and many others), then alphabetically by course title.

You might find some courses showing an award type '(Mod)', which indicates a combined degree that might be modular in design. A small number of courses have award type '(FYr)'. This indicates a 12-month foundation course, after which students can choose to apply for a degree course. In either case, you should contact the university or college for further details.

Generally speaking, when a courses comprises two or more subjects, the word used to connect the subjects indicates the make-up of the award: 'Subject A and Subject B' is a joint award, where both subjects carry equal weight; 'Subject A with Subject B' is a major/minor award, where Subject A accounts for at least 60 per cent of your study. If the title shows 'Subject A/Subject B', it may indicate that students can decide on the weighting of the subjects at the end of the first year. You should check with the university or college for full details.

Each entry in the UCAS sections shows the UCAS course code and the duration of the course. Where known, the entry contains details of the minimum qualification requirements for the course, as supplied to UCAS by the universities and colleges. Bear in mind that possessing the minimum qualifications does not guarantee acceptance to the course; there may be far more applicants than places. You may be asked to attend an interview, present a portfolio or sit an admissions test.

Before applying for any course, you are advised to contact the university or college to check any changes in entry requirements and to see if any new courses have come on stream since the data was approved for publication. To make this easy, each institution's entry starts with their address, email, phone and fax details, as well as their website address. You will also find it useful to check the entry profiles section, linked to Course Search at www.ucas.com.

guidance publications

SPECIAL OFFER
£5 OFF - £29.50 PLUS £5 P&P
RRP £34.50 plus £5 p&p

The Big Guide: The Official Universities & Colleges Entrance Guide & CD-ROM 2007

The essential resource for all students, advisers and careers libraries. The Big Guide is THE publication providing entry requirements for higher education in the UK. Fully updated for 2007, the Big Guide forms an important part of a student's research and can be used in all stages leading to the completion of their UCAS application. Includes the Entry Requirements CD-ROM.

The Entry Requirements CD-ROM 2007 Entry £15

This CD-ROM, which accompanies the Big Guide, is also available as a single item. Cost-effective and easy to use, this is the definitive guide to UK entry requirements, with all the qualifications that are in the Big Guide plus many more. You can search by subject, university or college, geographical region or course code.

'Progression to…' guides 2007 entry

A 'must have' for any school, college or careers library to give applicants the edge in some of the most competitive subject areas. Written by experts and packed with advice and guidance, including career options, entry routes, study tips, how to apply, profiles of courses and case studies, along with details of the courses and entry requirements. The courses are now organised by subject, allowing the user to quickly and easily identify and compare courses in their chosen area.

Art and Design £14.99

Economics, Finance and Accountancy £14.99

Engineering and Mathematics £14.99

Law £14.99

Order the complete Progression set (five titles) £59.99

Making the Most of University £9.99

Going to university and college can be a great experience, but it can also be hard work. This guide helps students develop the skills they need to take advantage of their time at university and college. Published by Trotman.

The Careers Directory £12.99

The one-stop guide to professional careers. Provides advice on the work involved, training opportunities, requirements and earnings for over 350 careers. Published by COA.

The Virgin Alternative Guide to British Universities 2007 £15.99

Uncovers every aspect of university life, not just in terms of rents and cost of living, but teaching quality, student satisfaction and where your course will lead you. Published by Virgin.

Students' Money Matters 2006 £14.99

Cutting through the jargon, this book offers advice on all the key money issues. Published by Trotman.

Scottish Guide 2007 £14.95

Lists the main degree and diploma courses at all the universities and higher education colleges in Scotland. Both Scottish and English entry requirements are given and advice is also included about choosing where to study, getting onto a course, finance and possible career areas.

The Times Good University Guide 2007 £15.99

Contains all the crucial facts and figures to help students to find the best university or college for the subject they want to study. Published by HarperCollins.

How to Complete Your UCAS Application 2007 Entry £11.99

Now in a larger format and redesigned for ease of use, this guide is a must for anyone applying to UCAS. Published by Trotman.

The Push Guide to Choosing a University £4.99

Explains the differences between higher education institutions and how they affect life as a student. Includes a questionnaire to help you find your ideal university or college. Published by Hodder Arnold. 3rd edition.

www.ucasbooks.com

ORDERING YOUR COPIES

ONLINE: www.ucasbooks.com
BY PHONE: 01242 544610
BY EMAIL: distribution@ucas.ac.uk
BY FAX: 01242 544806
BY POST: UCAS DISTRIBUTION, PO BOX 130, CHELTENHAM, GLOS GL52 3ZF

PAYMENT CAN BE IN THE FORM OF A CHEQUE, MADE PAYABLE TO UCAS ENTERPRISES LTD, OR CREDIT/DEBIT CARD DETAILS. WE ACCEPT VISA, DELTA, EUROCARD, MASTERCARD, SWITCH/MAESTRO, SOLO AND VISA ELECTRON. PLEASE QUOTE GTI WHEN PLACING YOUR ORDER.

P&P £3 FOR A SINGLE COPY ORDER AND £5 FOR A MULTIPLE COPY ORDER, EXCEPT THE BIG GUIDE WHERE THE CHARGE IS £5 PER ORDER.

MEDICINE

A20 THE UNIVERSITY OF ABERDEEN

UNIVERSITY OFFICE
KING'S COLLEGE
ABERDEEN AB24 3FX

t: +44 (0) 1224 273504 **f:** + 44 (0) 1224 272031
e: sras@abdn.ac.uk

// www.abdn.ac.uk/sras

A100 MB Medicine

Duration: 5FT Hon

Entry requirements: *GCE/AVCE:* AAB. *SQAH:* AAAAB. *SQAAH:* ABB. *IB:*
36. Interview required. Admissions Test required.

B32 THE UNIVERSITY OF BIRMINGHAM

EDGBASTON
BIRMINGHAM B15 2TT

t: 0121 414 5491 **f:** 0121 414 7159
e: admissions@bham.ac.uk

// www.bham.ac.uk

B900 BMedSc Medical Science

Duration: 3FT Hon

Entry requirements: *GCE/AVCE:* BBB. *SQAH:* BBBBB. *IB:* 32.

A100 MBChB Medicine (5 years)

Duration: 5FT Hon

Entry requirements: *GCE/AVCE:* AAB. *SQAH:* AAAAB. *IB:* 36. Interview
required.

A101 MBChB Medicine (Graduate Entry) (4 years)

Duration: 4FT Hon

Entry requirements: Interview required.

B56 THE UNIVERSITY OF BRADFORD

RICHMOND ROAD
BRADFORD
WEST YORKSHIRE BD7 1DP

t: 01274 233081 **f:** 01274 236260
e: course-enquiries@bradford.ac.uk

// www.bradford.ac.uk

B990 BSc Clinical Sciences

Duration: 3FT Hon

Entry requirements: *GCE/AVCE:* 280. *IB:* 30. Interview required.

B991 BSc Clinical Sciences/Medicine Foundation (Year 0)

Duration: 4FT Hon

Entry requirements: *GCE/AVCE:* 200. *IB:* 24. Interview required.

B74 BRIGHTON AND SUSSEX MEDICAL SCHOOL

UNIVERSITY OF BRIGHTON
MITHRAS HOUSE
LEWES ROAD
BRIGHTON BN2 4AT

t: 01273 600900 **f:** 01273 642825
e: medadmissions@bsms.ac.uk

// www.bsms.ac.uk

A100 BMBS Medicine

Duration: 5FT Hon

Entry requirements: *GCE/AVCE:* 340. *IB:* 37. Interview required.

B78 UNIVERSITY OF BRISTOL

UNDERGRADUATE ADMISSIONS OFFICE
SENATE HOUSE
TYNDALL AVENUE
BRISTOL BS8 1TH

t: 0117 928 9000 **f:** 0117 925 1424
e: admissions@bristol.ac.uk

// www.bristol.ac.uk

A104 MB Medicine - First MB,ChB (pre-medical) entry (6 years)

Duration: 6FT Hon

Entry requirements: *GCE/AVCE:* AAB. *SQAH:* AAAAA. *SQAAH:* AB. *IB:*
36. *BTEC ND:* DDM.

A100 MB Medicine - Second MB,ChB entry (5 years)

Duration: 5FT Hon

Entry requirements: *GCE/AVCE:* AAB. *SQAH:* AAAAA. *SQAAH:* AB. *IB:*
36.

A101 MBChB Medicine Graduate entry (4 years)

Duration: 4FT Hon

Entry requirements: Contact the institution for details.

C05 UNIVERSITY OF CAMBRIDGE

CAMBRIDGE ADMISSIONS OFFICE
FITZWILLIAM HOUSE
32 TRUMPINGTON STREET
CAMBRIDGE CB2 1QY

t: 01223 333 308 **f:** 01223 366 383
e: admissions@cam.ac.uk

// www.cam.ac.uk/admissions/undergraduate/

A101 MB Cambridge Graduate Course in Medicine

Duration: 4FT Hon

Entry requirements: Interview required.

A100 MB Medicine

Duration: 5FT/6FT Hon

Entry requirements: *GCE/AVCE:* AAA. *SQAAH:* AAA-AAB. Interview required. Admissions Test required.

C15 CARDIFF UNIVERSITY

PO BOX 927
30-36 NEWPORT ROAD
CARDIFF CF24 0DE

t: 029 2087 9999 f: 029 2087 6982
e: admissions@cardiff.ac.uk
// www.cardiff.ac.uk

A100 MBBCh Medicine (first-year entry)

Duration: 5FT Hon

Entry requirements: *GCE/AVCE:* 370. *SQAH:* AAAAB. *SQAAH:* AA. *IB:* 36. *BTEC NC:* DD. *BTEC ND:* DDD. Interview required. Admissions Test required.

A104 MBBCh Medicine (foundation course)

Duration: 6FT Hon

Entry requirements: *GCE/AVCE:* AAB. *SQAH:* AAAAB. *IB:* 36. *BTEC NC:* DD. *BTEC ND:* DDD. Interview required. Admissions Test required.

D65 UNIVERSITY OF DUNDEE

DUNDEE DD1 4HN

t: 01382 344160 f: 01382 348150
e: srs@dundee.ac.uk
// www.dundee.ac.uk

A100 MB Medicine

Duration: 5FT Hon

Entry requirements: *GCE/AVCE:* 360. *IB:* 34. Interview required.

A104 MB Medicine (Pre-medical year)

Duration: 6FT Hon

Entry requirements: *GCE/AVCE:* 360. *IB:* 34. Interview required.

E14 UNIVERSITY OF EAST ANGLIA

THE UNIVERSITY OF EAST ANGLIA
NORWICH NR4 7TJ

t: 01603 456161 f: 01603 458596
e: admissions@uea.ac.uk
// www.uea.ac.uk

A100 MBBS Medicine

Duration: 5FT Hon

Entry requirements: *GCE/AVCE:* 360. *IB:* 34. Interview required. Admissions Test required.

E56 THE UNIVERSITY OF EDINBURGH

STUDENT RECRUITMENT & ADMISSIONS
57 GEORGE SQUARE
EDINBURGH EH8 9JU

t: 0131 650 4360 f: 0131 651 1236
e: sra.enquiries@ed.ac.uk
// www.ed.ac.uk/studying/undergraduate/

A100 MBChB Medicine (5 years)

Duration: 5FT Hon

Entry requirements: *GCE/AVCE:* AAAb. *SQAH:* AAAAB. *IB:* 37. Admissions Test required.

A104 MBChB Medicine (6 years)

Duration: 6FT Hon

Entry requirements: *GCE/AVCE:* AAAb. *SQAH:* AAAAB. *IB:* 37. Admissions Test required.

B100 BSc Medical Sciences

Duration: 4FT Hon

Entry requirements: *GCE/AVCE:* BBB. *SQAH:* BBBB.

G28 UNIVERSITY OF GLASGOW

THE UNIVERSITY
GLASGOW G12 8QQ

t: 0141 330 4575 f: 0141 330 4045
e: admissions@gla.ac.uk
// www.gla.ac.uk

A100 MB Medicine

Duration: 5FT Hon

Entry requirements: *GCE/AVCE:* AAB. *SQAH:* AAAAB. *IB:* 36.

H75 HULL YORK MEDICAL SCHOOL

HYMS ADMISSIONS SECTION
ADMISSIONS & SCHOOLS LIAISON
UNIVERSITY OF YORK
HESLINGTON. YORK YO10 5DD

t: 0870 120 2323 f: 01904 433538
e: admissions@hyms.ac.uk
// www.hyms.ac.uk

A100 MBBS Medicine

Duration: 5FT Hon

Entry requirements: *GCE/AVCE:* AABb. *SQAH:* AAAAB. *SQAAH:* AB. *IB:* 36. Interview required. Admissions Test required.

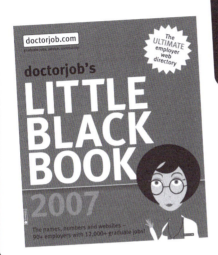
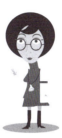
I50 IMPERIAL COLLEGE LONDON (UNIVERSITY OF LONDON)

REGISTRY: ADMISSIONS
SOUTH KENSINGTON CAMPUS
IMPERIAL COLLEGE LONDON
LONDON SW7 2AZ

t: 020 7594 8001 **f:** 020 7594 8004
e:

// www.imperial.ac.uk

A100 MBBS/BSc Medicine

Duration: 6FT Hon

Entry requirements: *GCE/AVCE:* AABb. *SQAAH:* AAB. Interview required. Admissions Test required.

K12 KEELE UNIVERSITY

KEELE UNIVERSITY
STAFFS ST5 5BG

t: 01782 584005 **f:** 01782 632343
e: undergraduate@keele.ac.uk

// www.keele.ac.uk

A100 MBChB Medicine

Duration: 5FT Hon

Entry requirements: *GCE/AVCE:* AAB. *SQAAH:* AAB. *IB:* 34. Interview required.

B900 MBChB Medicine with Health Foundation Year

Duration: 6FT Hon

Entry requirements: *GCE/AVCE:* AAB. *IB:* 26.

K60 KING'S COLLEGE LONDON (UNIVERSITY OF LONDON)

STRAND
LONDON WC2R 2LS

t: 020 7836 5454 **f:** 020 7836 1799
e: ucas.enquiries@kcl.ac.uk

// www.kcl.ac.uk

A101 MBBS6 Extended Medical Degree Programme (6 years)

Duration: 6FT Hon

Entry requirements: Contact the institution for details.

A100 MBBS Medicine (5 years)

Duration: 5FT Hon

Entry requirements: *GCE/AVCE:* AABc. *SQAAH:* AAB. *IB:* 36. Interview required.

A103 MBBS Medicine Conversion Entry Programme (6 years)

Duration: 6FT Hon

Entry requirements: *GCE/AVCE:* AABc. *SQAH:* AAABB. *SQAAH:* ABB. *IB:* 35. Interview required.

A102 MBBS Medicine Graduate/Professional Entry Programme (4 years)

Duration: 4FT Hon

Entry requirements: Admissions Test required.

A104 MBBS Medicine Maxfax Entry Programme (MFDS candidates only/4 years)

Duration: 4FT Hon

Entry requirements: Interview required.

L14 LANCASTER UNIVERSITY
THE UNIVERSITY
LANCASTER
LANCASHIRE LA1 4YW
t: 01524 65201 f: 01524 846243
e: ugadmissions@lancaster.ac.uk
// www.lancs.ac.uk

A900 CertHE Pre-Medical Studies

Duration: 1FT Cer

Entry requirements: *GCE/AVCE:* BBB-BBC. *SQAH:* BBBBB-BBBCC.

L23 UNIVERSITY OF LEEDS
THE UNIVERSITY
LEEDS LS2 9JT
t: 0113 343 3999 f: 0113 343 3877
e: admissions@adm.leeds.ac.uk
// www.leeds.ac.uk

A100 MBChB Medicine

Duration: 5FT Hon

Entry requirements: *GCE/AVCE:* AAB. *SQAH:* AAAAB. *IB:* 36. Admissions Test required.

L34 UNIVERSITY OF LEICESTER
UNIVERSITY ROAD
LEICESTER LE1 7RH
t: 0116 252 5281 f: 0116 252 2447
e: admissions@le.ac.uk
// www.le.ac.uk

A101 MBChB Medicine (4 years)

Duration: 4FT Hon

Entry requirements: Interview required. Admissions Test required.

A100 MBChB Medicine (5 years)

Duration: 5FT Hon

Entry requirements: *GCE/AVCE:* AAB. *SQAH:* AAAAA. *SQAAH:* AAB. *IB:* 36. *BTEC ND:* DDD. Interview required. Admissions Test required.

L41 THE UNIVERSITY OF LIVERPOOL
SENATE HOUSE
ABERCROMBY SQUARE
LIVERPOOL L69 3BX
t: 0151 794 2000 f: 0151 708 6502
e: ugrecruitment@liv.ac.uk
// www.liv.ac.uk

B900 BSc Life Sciences applicable to Medicine

Duration: 3FT Hon

Entry requirements: *GCE/AVCE:* 280-300. *SQAH:* BBBBC. *SQAAH:* BBC. *BTEC ND:* MMM.

A100 MBChB Medicine

Duration: 5FT Hon

Entry requirements: *GCE/AVCE:* AABb. *SQAH:* AAAAA-AAABB. *SQAAH:* AA. *IB:* 38. Interview required.

A101 MBChB Medicine (Graduate Entry)

Duration: 4FT Hon

Entry requirements: Interview required.

A105 MBChB Medicine (based at Lancaster University)

Duration: 5FT Hon

Entry requirements: Refer to institution.

M20 THE UNIVERSITY OF MANCHESTER
THE UNIVERSITY OF MANCHESTER
OXFORD ROAD
MANCHESTER M13 9PL
t: 0161 275 2077 f: 0161 275 2106
e: ug.admissions@manchester.ac.uk
// www.manchester.ac.uk

A106 MBChB Medicine (5 years)

Duration: 5FT Hon

Entry requirements: *GCE/AVCE:* AAB. *SQAAH:* AAB. *IB:* 35. Interview required. Admissions Test required.

A104 MBChB Medicine (6 years including foundation year)

Duration: 6FT Hon

Entry requirements: *GCE/AVCE:* ABB. *SQAH:* AAABB. *SQAAH:* ABB. Interview required. Admissions Test required.

N21 UNIVERSITY OF NEWCASTLE UPON TYNE

6 KENSINGTON TERRACE
NEWCASTLE UPON TYNE NE1 7RU

t: 0191 222 5594 **f:** 0191 222 6143
e: enquiries@ncl.ac.uk

// www.ncl.ac.uk

A101 MBBS Medicine (Accelerated Programme, Graduate Entry)

Duration: 4FT Hon

Entry requirements: Interview required.

A106 MBBS Medicine (stage 1 entry)

Duration: 5FT Hon

Entry requirements: *GCE/AVCE:* AAA. *SQAH:* AAAAA. *IB:* 38. Interview required. Admissions Test required.

N84 THE UNIVERSITY OF NOTTINGHAM

THE ADMISSIONS OFFICE
E FLOOR, PORTLAND BUILDING
UNIVERSITY OF NOTTINGHAM
UNIVERSITY PARK. NOTTINGHAM NG7 2RD

t: 0115 951 5151 **f:** 0115 951 4668
e:

// www.nottingham.ac.uk

A100 BMBS Medicine

Duration: 5FT Hon

Entry requirements: *GCE/AVCE:* AAB. *SQAAH:* AAB. *IB:* 38. Interview required. Admissions Test required.

A101 BMBS Medicine (Graduate Entry)

Duration: 4FT Hon

Entry requirements: Interview required. Admissions Test required.

O33 OXFORD UNIVERSITY

OXFORD COLLEGES ADMISSIONS OFFICE
WELLINGTON SQUARE
OXFORD OX1 2JD

t: 01865 288000 **f:** 01865 270708
e: undergraduate.admissions@ox.ac.uk

// www.admissions.ox.ac.uk

A100 BMBCh Medicine

Duration: 6FT Hon

Entry requirements: *GCE/AVCE:* AAA. *SQAH:* AAAAA-AAAAB. *SQAAH:* AAA. *IB:* 38. Interview required. Admissions Test required.

A101 BMBCh4 Medicine (Fast-track, Graduate Entry only)

Duration: 4FT Hon

Entry requirements: *IB:* 38. Interview required. Admissions Test required.

P37 PENINSULA MEDICAL SCHOOL

PENINSULA MEDICAL SCHOOL
TAMAR SCIENCE PARK
RESEARCH WAY
PLYMOUTH PL6 8BU

t: 01752 247334 **f:** 01752 517842
e: medadmissions@pms.ac.uk

// www.pms.ac.uk

A100 BMBS Medicine

Duration: 5FT Hon

Entry requirements: *GCE/AVCE:* 370-400. *IB:* 38. *BTEC NC:* DD. *BTEC ND:* DDD. Interview required. Admissions Test required.

Q50 QUEEN MARY, UNIVERSITY OF LONDON

MILE END ROAD
LONDON E1 4NS

t: 0800 376 1800 **f:** 020 7882 5500
e: admissions@qmul.ac.uk

// www.qmul.ac.uk

A100 MBBS Medicine

Duration: 5FT Hon

Entry requirements: *GCE/AVCE:* AAB. *SQAH:* AAA. *SQAAH:* BB. *IB:* 36.

A101 MBBS Medicine (Graduate Entry)

Duration: 4FT Hon

Entry requirements: *IB:* 36. Admissions Test required.

Q75 QUEEN'S UNIVERSITY BELFAST

UNIVERSITY ROAD
BELFAST BT7 1NN

t: 028 9097 5081 **f:** 028 9097 5137
e: admissions@qub.ac.uk

// www.qub.ac.uk

A100 MB Medicine

Duration: 5FT Hon

Entry requirements: *GCE/AVCE:* AAAa. *SQAH:* AAAAA. *SQAAH:* AAA. *IB:* 37.

S18 THE UNIVERSITY OF SHEFFIELD

9 NORTHUMBERLAND ROAD
SHEFFIELD S10 2TT

t: 0114 222 2000 **f:** 0114 222 8032
e: ug.admissions@sheffield.ac.uk

// www.sheffield.ac.uk

A104 MBChB Medicine (Foundation Year)

Duration: 6FT Hon

Entry requirements: *GCE/AVCE:* AAB. *SQAH:* AAAAB. *SQAAH:* AB. *IB:* 34.

A100 MBChB Medicine (Phase One)

Duration: 5FT Hon

Entry requirements: *GCE/AVCE:* AAB. *SQAH:* AAAAB. *SQAAH:* AB. *IB:* 34.

S27 UNIVERSITY OF SOUTHAMPTON

HIGHFIELD
SOUTHAMPTON SO17 1BJ

t: 023 8059 5000 f: 023 8059 3037
e: admissions@soton.ac.uk

// www.soton.ac.uk

A101 BM Medicine - Graduate entry (4 year)

Duration: 4FT Hon

Entry requirements: Contact the institution for details.

A102 BM Medicine - Widening access (6 year) incl Foundation

Duration: 6FT Hon

Entry requirements: Interview required. Admissions Test required.

A100 BM Medicine (5 year)

Duration: 5FT Hon

Entry requirements: *GCE/AVCE:* AAB. *SQAH:* AAAAB. *SQAAH:* AB. *IB:* 36. Admissions Test required.

S36 UNIVERSITY OF ST ANDREWS

ADMISSIONS OFFICE
79 NORTH STREET
ST ANDREWS
FIFE KY16 9AJ

t: 01334 462150 f: 01334 463388
e: admissions@st-andrews.ac.uk

// www.st-and.ac.uk

A100 BSc Medicine (BSc Honours)

Duration: 3FT Hon

Entry requirements: *GCE/AVCE:* AAB. *SQAH:* AAABB. *IB:* 36.

S49 ST GEORGE'S, UNIVERSITY OF LONDON (FORMERLY ST GEORGE'S HOSPITAL MEDICAL SCHOOL)

CRANMER TERRACE
LONDON SW17 0RE

t: 020 8725 5201 / 0499 f: 020 8725 2734
e: see below

// www.sgul.ac.uk

A100 MBBS Medicine

Duration: 5FT Hon

Entry requirements: *GCE/AVCE:* AABb-BBCb. *SQAH:* AAAAA-BBBBB. *SQAAH:* AAA-AAB. Interview required. Admissions Test required.

A101 MBBS Medicine (4-year Graduate Entry)

Duration: 4FT Hon

Entry requirements: Interview required. Admissions Test required.

A103 FYr Foundation for Medicine

Duration: 1FT FYr

Entry requirements: Interview required.

S93 UNIVERSITY OF WALES SWANSEA

SINGLETON PARK
SWANSEA SA2 8PP

t: 01792 295111 f: 01792 295110
e: admissions@swansea.ac.uk

// www.swansea.ac.uk

A101 MBBCh Medicine

Duration: 4FT Hon

Entry requirements: Interview required. Admissions Test required.

U80 UNIVERSITY COLLEGE LONDON (UNIVERSITY OF LONDON)

UCL
GOWER STREET
LONDON WC1E 6BT

t: 020 7679 3000 f: 020 7679 3001
e:

// www.ucl.ac.uk

A100 MBBS Medicine (6 years)

Duration: 6FT Hon

Entry requirements: *GCE/AVCE:* AABe. *SQAAH:* AAB. *IB:* 36. Admissions Test required.

W20 THE UNIVERSITY OF WARWICK

UNIVERSITY OF WARWICK
COVENTRY CV4 8UW

t: 024 7652 3723 f: 024 7652 4649
e: ugadmissions@warwick.ac.uk

// www.warwick.ac.uk

A101 MBChB Medicine MBChB

Duration: 4FT Hon

Entry requirements: Interview required. Admissions Test required.

DENTISTRY

B32 THE UNIVERSITY OF BIRMINGHAM

EDGBASTON
BIRMINGHAM B15 2TT
t: 0121 414 5491 f: 0121 414 7159
e: admissions@bham.ac.uk
// www.bham.ac.uk

A200 BDS Dentistry (5 years)

Duration: 5FT Hon

Entry requirements: *GCE/AVCE:* AAB-ABB. *SQAH:* AAAAB. *SQAAH:* AAB. *IB:* 36. Interview required.

B78 UNIVERSITY OF BRISTOL

UNDERGRADUATE ADMISSIONS OFFICE
SENATE HOUSE
TYNDALL AVENUE
BRISTOL BS8 1TH
t: 0117 928 9000 f: 0117 925 1424
e: admissions@bristol.ac.uk
// www.bristol.ac.uk

A204 BDS Dentistry - First BDS (pre-dental) entry (6 years)

Duration: 6FT Hon

Entry requirements: *GCE/AVCE:* AAB. *SQAH:* AAAAB. *SQAAH:* AB. *IB:* 36. *BTEC ND:* DDD.

A206 BDS Dentistry - Second BDS entry (5 years)

Duration: 5FT Hon

Entry requirements: *GCE/AVCE:* AAB. *SQAH:* AAAAB. *SQAAH:* AB. *IB:* 36. *BTEC ND:* DDD.

C15 CARDIFF UNIVERSITY

PO BOX 927
30-36 NEWPORT ROAD
CARDIFF CF24 0DE
t: 029 2087 9999 f: 029 2087 6982
e: admissions@cardiff.ac.uk
// www.cardiff.ac.uk

A200 BDS BDS (first-year entry)

Duration: 5FT Hon

Entry requirements: *GCE/AVCE:* AAB. *SQAAH:* BB. *IB:* 34. Interview required. Admissions Test required.

A204 BDS BDS (foundation course)

Duration: 6FT Hon

Entry requirements: *GCE/AVCE:* AAB. *SQAH:* ABBBB. *IB:* 34. *BTEC ND:* DDD. Interview required. Admissions Test required.

D65 UNIVERSITY OF DUNDEE

DUNDEE DD1 4HN
t: 01382 344160 f: 01382 348150
e: srs@dundee.ac.uk
// www.dundee.ac.uk

A200 BDS Dentistry

Duration: 5FT Hon

Entry requirements: *GCE/AVCE:* 360. *SQAH:* AAAAA. Interview required.

A204 BDS Dentistry (Pre-dental year)

Duration: 6FT Hon

Entry requirements: *GCE/AVCE:* 360. *SQAH:* AAAAA. Interview required.

G28 UNIVERSITY OF GLASGOW

THE UNIVERSITY
GLASGOW G12 8QQ
t: 0141 330 4575 f: 0141 330 4045
e: admissions@gla.ac.uk
// www.gla.ac.uk

A200 BDS Dentistry

Duration: 5FT Hon

Entry requirements: *GCE/AVCE:* AAB. *SQAH:* AAAAB. *IB:* 34. Interview required. Admissions Test required. Portfolio required.

K60 KING'S COLLEGE LONDON (UNIVERSITY OF LONDON)

STRAND
LONDON WC2R 2LS
t: 020 7836 5454 f: 020 7836 1799
e: ucas.enquiries@kcl.ac.uk
// www.kcl.ac.uk

A205 BDS Dentistry (5 years)

Duration: 5FT Hon

Entry requirements: *GCE/AVCE:* AABc. *SQAAH:* ABB. *IB:* 36. Interview required. Admissions Test required.

A203 BDS Dentistry Conversion Entry Programme (6 years)

Duration: 6FT Hon

Entry requirements: *GCE/AVCE:* AABc. *SQAH:* ABBBB. *SQAAH:* ABB. *IB:* 35. Interview required.

A202 BDS Dentistry Graduate/Professional Entry Programme (4 years)

Duration: 4FT Hon

Entry requirements: Interview required.

L23 UNIVERSITY OF LEEDS

THE UNIVERSITY
LEEDS LS2 9JT

t: 0113 343 3999 f: 0113 343 3877
e: admissions@adm.leeds.ac.uk

// www.leeds.ac.uk

A200 BChD Dentistry

Duration: 5FT Hon

Entry requirements: *GCE/AVCE:* AAB. *IB:* 35.

L41 THE UNIVERSITY OF LIVERPOOL

SENATE HOUSE
ABERCROMBY SQUARE
LIVERPOOL L69 3BX

t: 0151 794 2000 f: 0151 708 6502
e: ugrecruitment@liv.ac.uk

// www.liv.ac.uk

A200 BDS Dental Surgery

Duration: 5FT Hon

Entry requirements: *GCE/AVCE:* 340-390. *SQAH:* AAAAB. *SQAAH:* AAB. *IB:* 36. *BTEC ND:* DDD. Interview required.

A201 BDS Dental Surgery (Graduate Entry)

Duration: 4FT Hon

Entry requirements: Contact the institution for details.

M20 THE UNIVERSITY OF MANCHESTER

THE UNIVERSITY OF MANCHESTER
OXFORD ROAD
MANCHESTER M13 9PL

t: 0161 275 2077 f: 0161 275 2106
e: ug.admissions@manchester.ac.uk

// www.manchester.ac.uk

A206 BDS Dentistry (BDS first-year entry)

Duration: 5FT Hon

Entry requirements: *GCE/AVCE:* AAB. *SQAH:* AAAAB. *SQAAH:* AB. *IB:* 35. Interview required. Admissions Test required.

A204 BDS Dentistry (BDS pre-dental year entry)

Duration: 6FT Hon

Entry requirements: *GCE/AVCE:* ABB. *SQAH:* AABBB. *SQAAH:* AB. *IB:* 33. Interview required. Admissions Test required.

N21 UNIVERSITY OF NEWCASTLE UPON TYNE

6 KENSINGTON TERRACE
NEWCASTLE UPON TYNE NE1 7RU

t: 0191 222 5594 f: 0191 222 6143
e: enquiries@ncl.ac.uk

// www.ncl.ac.uk

A206 BDS Dentistry

Duration: 5FT Hon

Entry requirements: *GCE/AVCE:* AAB. *SQAH:* AAAAB. *IB:* 35. Interview required. Admissions Test required.

P37 PENINSULA MEDICAL SCHOOL

PENINSULA MEDICAL SCHOOL
TAMAR SCIENCE PARK
RESEARCH WAY
PLYMOUTH PL6 8BU

t: 01752 247334 f: 01752 517842
e: medadmissions@pms.ac.uk

// www.pms.ac.uk

A201 BDS Dentistry Graduate Entry (4 years)

Duration: 4FT Hon

Entry requirements: Interview required.

Q50 QUEEN MARY, UNIVERSITY OF LONDON

MILE END ROAD
LONDON E1 4NS

t: 0800 376 1800 f: 020 7882 5500
e: admissions@qmul.ac.uk

// www.qmul.ac.uk

A200 BDS Dentistry

Duration: 5FT Hon

Entry requirements: *GCE/AVCE:* AAB. *SQAH:* AAA. *SQAAH:* BB. *IB:* 36.

A201 BDS Dentistry (Graduate Entry)

Duration: 4FT Hon

Entry requirements: Contact the institution for details.

Q75 QUEEN'S UNIVERSITY BELFAST

UNIVERSITY ROAD
BELFAST BT7 1NN

t: 028 9097 5081 f: 028 9097 5137
e: admissions@qub.ac.uk

// www.qub.ac.uk

A200 BDS Dentistry

Duration: 5FT Hon

Entry requirements: *GCE/AVCE:* AAAa. *SQAH:* AAAAA. *SQAAH:* AAA. *IB:* 37.

S18 THE UNIVERSITY OF SHEFFIELD

9 NORTHUMBERLAND ROAD
SHEFFIELD S10 2TT

t: 0114 222 2000 f: 0114 222 8032
e: ug.admissions@sheffield.ac.uk

// www.sheffield.ac.uk

A200 BDS Dentistry

Duration: 5FT Hon

Entry requirements: *GCE/AVCE:* AAB-AAab. *SQAH:* AAAAB. *SQAAH:* AB. *IB:* 33.

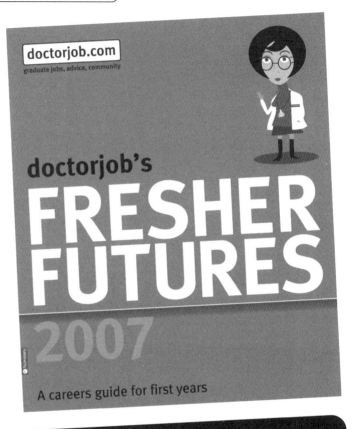
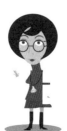

Medicine profiles

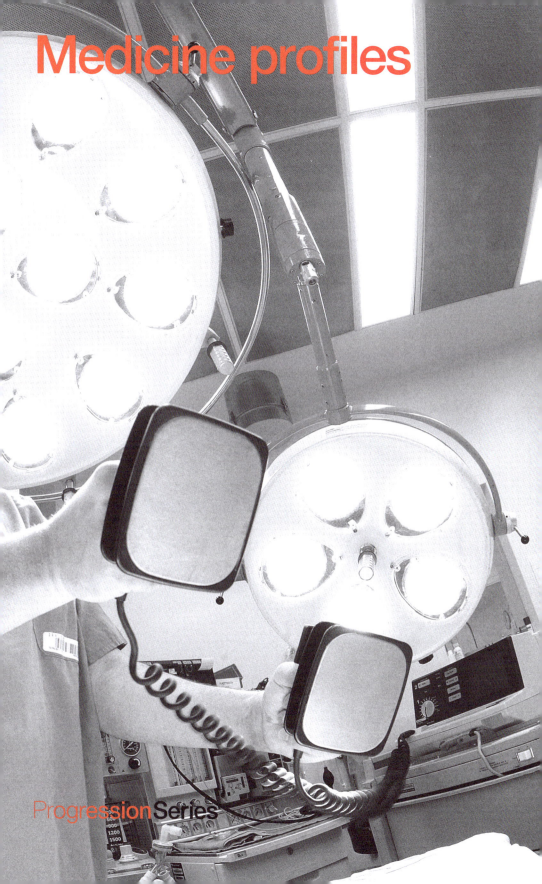

Birmingham B32

A100

DESIRABLE SKILLS/QUALITIES AT ENTRY

Interpersonal skills

No offers are made without an interview. At interview it is important that applicants demonstrate they are well-informed about, and strongly motivated towards, a career in medicine, and possess the other qualities required of a doctor. The interview is competitive. The minimum academic entry requirements are listed on the medical school website.

Learning skills

With tutorial guidance, students need to be able to direct and develop their own learning strategies and skills. They should be self-motivated, good at time management and able to withstand the unique stresses of an undergraduate medical course.

Information technology

Although students will be taught many aspects of information technology, some experience in word processing and spreadsheets is an advantage.

SKILLS DEVELOPED ON THE COURSE

Learning skills

Throughout their training, students are encouraged to develop and practise the independent and self-directed learning skills vital to a doctor. This personal commitment to learning is supported by expert lectures, small group teaching and supervised clinical experience. Part of the training in research and evidence-based medicine is learning to access the medical school's considerable library and computer-based learning resources.

Information technology

The medical school has an up-to-date computer/IT suite. All students develop the skills necessary for information retrieval by accessing references and databases. Competence will also be developed in data collection and analysis.

Interpersonal skills

Students learn about communication skills, the biological and behavioural sciences, ethics, law and public health as they apply to the practice of medicine. The clinical sciences are taught as an integral part of a programme of varied clinical experience. In short, every opportunity is provided to develop the knowledge, skills and attitudes needed as a foundation for practice and continuing professional development.

Bristol B78

A106

ABOUT THE COURSE

- A degree in medicine equips students for a professional career as a doctor. The programme has a strong emphasis on integrated teaching, early clinical experience, and a strong science base, with extensive tutorial group support.

- It is divided into three phases: in phase 1, students experience patient contact straightaway and learn general principles underlying behavioural science and basic medical science (two terms); phase 2 comprises formal teaching on the body systems with full-time clinical attachments in year three (two years); phase 3 is clinical training, covering more specialist areas (two years).

SPECIAL FEATURES

- Initially, most medical teaching takes place in the School of Medical Sciences itself, whose excellent facilities are in the main university precinct. Teaching also takes place in the numerous NHS Trust hospitals and general practices in the city.

- During years 3 to 5, students attend teaching at a clinical academy – half the year is spent in an academy in Bristol and the other half is based at a 'regional' academy. Across the three clinical years, students are placed at as many of the different academies as possible to provide the widest possible experience. This allows them to engage fully in the ongoing clinical activities across the region, and to take the chance of training alongside other healthcare professionals.

WHAT SKILLS, QUALITIES AND EXPERIENCE
DO I NEED?

- The programme is strong in research-informed teaching. All the departments in the Faculty of Medicine and Dentistry and in the Faculty of Medical and Veterinary Sciences are internationally renowned for their research, so students are taught by people who are world experts in their fields. The university's research strengths include neuroscience, cancer biology, and immunology.

- At the end of year 2, or exceptionally year 3, students may be able to intercalate an extra year in order to study for an honours BSc degree. Subjects available include anatomical science, biochemistry, bioethics, pathology and microbiology, pharmacology, physiology and neuroscience. Some financial assistance may be available for this extra year.

- The programme includes a series of student-centred projects, known as 'student-selected components', involving studying particular subject areas in depth, as well as offering the opportunity to study modern languages.

- There is the option of studying abroad (elective study) for two months in the final year. In addition, the Bristol Medical School was a pioneer of the European Credit Transfer Scheme, and offers the opportunity of spending three to six months at a participating European medical school in year 3 and receiving credit for academic work successfully undertaken there.

- Medicine is a profession that inspires, but also requires commitment. Students should use their UCAS personal statement to explain their reasons for wanting to study the course and why they would make a good doctor. Applicants need to be able to demonstrate that they fully grasp what a medical career involves, and are aware of current developments.

- An excellent academic profile, with predicted AAB at A level, and a majority of GCSE grades at A/A* is necessary.

- Science underpins most clinical skills. It is important to enjoy, as well as understand, the basic sciences. Applicants are expected to have read outside their A level subjects and be aware of current scientific issues.

- The UCAS personal statement needs to reveal the effort applicants have made to find out what it would be like to work as a doctor. This does not necessarily mean medically-related work experience, such as shadowing a GP or consultant, as this can be difficult to obtain under the age of 18. However, caring experience, whether medically-related or not (for example, a hospital, an old people's home), is an advantage. An insight into medicine and healthcare gained from general reading is expected. It might also be useful to attend medical careers conferences, or to talk to doctors or current medical students.

- Good communication skills are essential. Doctors need to be able to explain complex information simply and coherently. Some knowledge of a European language is also useful for those who wish to participate in European exchanges.

- A logical mind is needed to formulate questions and solve problems.

- Self-motivation is needed. Can you set your own goals and show independence of thought? Students also need to be able to work well in a team and be prepared to work long hours.

- A good doctor needs to have a strong interest in human affairs, and a concern for the welfare of others, to reassure people and put them at their ease.

- Bristol is also interested in extra-curricular activities, and general interests, especially where this illustrates engagement with the wider community. The concern is not with what applicants do, but that they use their spare time to advantage.

- Doctors must develop a high standard of professional responsibility, so applicants need to demonstrate that they are reliable and conscientious.

Dundee D65

A100

- Students follow a problem-orientated, student-centred and community-based course.

- Real clinical experience is available from from year 1 with direct patient contact.

- There is a choice of what to study from a wide range of SSC (Student Selected Components) modules and students can even propose their own. SSC modules form one third of the course.

- Students can choose from a range of clinical attachments in Dundee, Tayside and elsewhere in Scotland and the UK. In the final year, there is the opportunity to travel anywhere in the world to undertake a period of elective study.

Two components, a common core and SSCs, provide depth and breadth in an exciting curriculum.

CORE

The integrated, systematic course is under constant review to improve and develop its design. Dundee is working towards closer integration between phase 1 (year 1) and phase 2 (years 2 and 3) to ensure that the content truly supports the outcomes and tasks required in phase 3.

PHASES 1 AND 2 (YEARS 1-3)

The course begins with an introduction to the outcomes. The main component of the first three years is an integrated body systems course dealing with normal and abnormal structure, function and behaviour.

Contributions come from anatomy, biochemistry, physiology, pharmacology and behavioural sciences, and there is a systematic study of clinical medicine, including health promotion and disease prevention. Early contact with real and simulated patients is promoted in the learning environments of community, hospital ward and clinical skills centre.

Blocks of study cover every system of the body. This ensures that by the end of year 3, students have a range of clinical experiences, skills and knowledge on which to proceed to phase 3.

PHASE 3 (YEARS 4 AND 5)

Students further advance their understanding of medicine in the context of a series of clinical attachments. Learning is centred upon 100 clinical tasks or problems, which bring together experiences gained in the attachments. The problems are designed to help students master the competencies required when they take up pre-registration foundation posts. During the fifth year, there is the opportunity of an attachment to the clinical units where foundation posts are undertaken after graduation.

The core component of the programme emphasises the competencies necessary for a newly qualified doctor to work in the hospital or community.

STUDENT SELECTED COMPONENTS (SSCS)

Flexibility is key to the programme. SSCs comprise approximately one third of the undergraduate course. They cover the following.

- A more in-depth study of the core, eg 'Surgery Beyond the Core'.

- Additional topics related to the core, eg 'Sports Medicine'.

- Other topics related to medicine, eg 'Human Rights' and 'Travel Medicine'.

- Additional topics, eg computing and languages.

They allow you to study topics of particular interest that can help students choose a branch of medicine as a career. They encourage the development of abilities in self-study, critical thinking and problem-solving.

Students construct their own SSCs or choose from a wide selection of modules. Some are undertaken abroad, eg the seven-week elective in phase 3. Others are mini-research projects that may be published in scientific journals.

Imperial I50

A100

Imperial's Faculty of Medicine was established in 1997, bringing together the major west London Medical Schools into one institution. The faculty is one of Europe's largest medical institutions in terms of staff and student population and its research income.

Its six-year undergraduate course is structured to meet the requirements of the General Medical Council Education Committee, as set out in the *Tomorrow's Doctors* report, and incorporates a BSc degree designed to take full advantage of the range of opportunities in science, engineering and management available at Imperial College.

The course aims to produce exceptional medical practitioners and future leaders of the profession. This is achieved through its first class teaching and internationally competitive research. Students acquire

the scientific knowledge, clinical skills and professional attitudes required for the care of patients and for research.

Teaching for much of the first part of the course is based at the South Kensington campus in the Sir Alexander Fleming building. This purpose-built facility is designed for learning medicine in the 21st century. It employs the latest technology, including fibre-optic video links with hospital sites, multidisciplinary teaching and computer laboratories, and an extensive IT network for supporting computer-assisted learning. Students have access to the central library facilities on the South Kensington campus.

TEACHING HOSPITALS

Imperial has access to a wide range of the clinical facilities at the Chelsea and Westminster Hospital, St Mary's Hospital, Paddington, Northwick Park Hospital, Harrow and the Charing Cross Hospital in Fulham.

Students receive additional training at other hospitals across west London. Students may live in for short periods at several hospitals outside London.

A large number of GP practices offer students valuable community and primary care experience.

MEDICINE

The course structure retains some elements of traditional medical courses whilst integrating clinical experience with the development of knowledge.

The course has the following additional distinctive features.

- It is a six-year course.
- All students will graduate with both an MBBS and a BSc degree.
- It combines the best of the traditional medical courses with more emphasis on communication skills, medical ethics and law, and information technology.

Leeds L23

A100

The course promotes learning that is integrated, provides early contact with patients and takes place in the community as well as in hospital. It uses a range of teaching and learning approaches consistent with producing self-directed students capable of continuing to learn. The needs of students, patients and the community are put to the fore.

Doctors need a variety of skills to deal with patients and to diagnose and treat their ills. These include clinical skills, communication skills and the ability to find the right information and apply it in a medical situation. Leeds aims to ensure graduates are:

- clinically competent;
- able to see patients as complete persons and have a holistic and ethically-based approach, including the capacity to understand and manage a patient's problems, in a family and social context, as well as in hospital;

- culturally tolerant, treating all patients and colleagues with respect, dignity and sensitivity;
- skilled at teamwork;
- prepared for continual learning;
- competent in medical information management;
- able to contribute to the continuing development of Medicine.

The medical curriculum is under continuous review and conforms to the recommendations in *Tomorrow's Doctors,* published by the General Medical Council.

- Basic sciences and clinical topics are integrated and based on systems, ie in 'nutrition and energy' students study anatomical, physiological, biochemical and clinical aspects.

- They meet patients from the start of the course.

- Students receive a balance of clinical experience between primary and community care, and hospitals.

- They develop skills in information technology and communication necessary throughout a medical career.

- Students practise clinical skills, for example, giving injections or setting up a drip, in one of the clinical skills centres to improve their skills before trying them on patients.

- The assessments, both theoretical and practical, are designed to help students learn and measure their competence.

- Students can also choose a range of topics outside the core throughout the course. These are known as student selected components (SSCs). For example, in the second year, it is possible to spend two weeks with the West Yorkshire Police or learn a new language. In the third year, there is a five-week block with over 200 topics to choose from, or they even have the option to design their own course.

The curriculum is divided into three phases.

PHASE I – PREPARING FOR CLINICAL PRACTICE

This phase is made up of a group of integrated core units (ICUs), which cover the initial groundwork needed in scientific and medical topics to allow students to start to develop as doctors.

Personal and professional development

This ICU runs throughout the first three years. The unit is designed to help students evaluate their capabilities and personal effectiveness, be skilled at teamwork and

be prepared for a lifetime of learning by being able to critically assess scientific information. It underpins all the other courses by providing a framework to initiate a personal development plan.

Individuals and populations

This unit runs over two years and aims to introduce students to health and illness within and across populations. Students gain a basic understanding of human experience and behaviour in health and illness, including the use of alternative and complementary therapies and the ways in which people and societies organise themselves to deal with the consequences of illness. They also receive an introduction to the UK National Health Service.

Nutrition and energy

In this first-year unit, students study the digestive system and develop an understanding of digestion, absorption, storage and utilisation of food in health and disease. Clinical lectures and videos link the basic science with conditions commonly encountered in clinical practice, such as diabetes, malabsorption, obesity and eating disorders.

Biomedical sciences

This two-year unit provides a foundation of scientific knowledge and principles which you will be able to relate to current medical practice and future advances. Clinicians provide sessions that link the basic scientific principles to their practice with patients.

Transport

This first-year unit looks at the processes and control mechanisms involved in maintaining homeostasis within the cardio-respiratory and renal systems of the body.

Control and movement

This second-year unit studies the nervous and musculo-skeletal system to understand the normal structure and function, and the nature of some of the common pathologies.

Students learn how this basic knowledge is related to the practice of clinical medicine, such as basic neurological examination.

Life cycle

This third-year unit provides an appreciation of the continuum of change from conception to death and the effects of these changes on the body, on the individual and on society.

Students recognise the application of the principles in differing clinical settings and consider the ethical, social and cultural issues within each clinical situation.

Patient evaluation: essential clinical skills and laboratory science

This second-year unit is an opportunity to start developing practical clinical skills in the assessment and investigation of patients.

The course takes students onto hospital wards and into general practices to develop history-taking and examining skills. In the second half of the third year, four days a week are spent with a hospital team or in a general practice either in Leeds or surrounding districts.

PHASE II – CLINICAL PRACTICE IN CONTEXT

Having spent phase I acquiring generic clinical skills, students then meet patients with more particular needs. The course has three sections for which students take one section for 15 weeks and then change to one of the other two.

- Paediatrics, obstetrics and gynaecology
- Primary care, psychiatry and public health
- Medical and surgical specialities

PHASE III – BECOMING A DOCTOR, ENHANCING CLINICAL COMPETENCE

For the first part of the fifth year, students have a period of 10 weeks of elective study, which can be undertaken anywhere. Students often go abroad to gain clinical experience or carry out a research project in different hospital settings.

After returning to Leeds and an introductory week in October, students take a rotation of five four-week placements (integrated clinical attachments) in Leeds and other Yorkshire hospitals and in general practices.

Most placements have a major theme of a common condition or disease and timetables are designed to present different aspects, both medical and surgical, and to gain hands-on experience. The year is designed to prepare students to become pre-registration house officers (PRHOs) in the first foundation year.

After written and practical examinations, four weeks are spent 'shadowing' the pre-registration house jobs.

Leicester L34

A100

The Leicester Medical School runs a five-year MBChB and a four-year accelerated MBChB course for graduates of health sciences. Both curricula are highly integrated, 'horizontally' so that disciplines within medicine are learned together, and 'vertically' in that clinical work and relevance are introduced from the beginning. All are divided into two phases. Phase 1 lays foundations that are built upon by full-time clinical work in phase 2. Phase 1 lasts two and a half years for the five-year course, and one and a half years for the four-year course. Phase 2 is exactly the same for both curricula.

PHASE 1 – LAYING THE FOUNDATIONS

Whichever course they take, students develop the knowledge, skills and attitudes necessary to communicate with patients, examine them and interpret their observations. Students take a core course, plus special study modules (SSMs), in which topics are chosen to suit individual interests and aspirations. Phase 1 is modular, over five semesters for the five-year course and three semesters for the four-year course.

Clinical Skills

Much of the time in phase 1 is spent in direct clinical work. Students meet patients very early on. Clinical and communication skills are developed in a structured way, first by attachment to a family, and work with volunteers and actors simulating patients, and then by work with real patients in hospital.

Medical Sciences

Students learn medical sciences through integrated, interdisciplinary modules. Applied subjects like pathology, microbiology and pharmacology are introduced very early, to make clear normal and abnormal function.

Social and Behavioural Medicine

Doctors must be aware that patients have social and psychological dimensions to their lives that affect the kind of illness from which they suffer. Therefore many modules emphasise the behavioural and social dimensions in clinical practice. Students learn about the full range of services for patients in need by working in multi-agency community centres.

Learning How to Learn

Medicine requires a commitment to lifelong learning. The aim is to develop self-directed learning. Core modules in phase 1 have few lectures, much more group work and learning by problem solving. There is lots of time for self study and, guided by the course objectives, students learn how to organise their own work.

Learning to Integrate

However integrated the curriculum, the subjects relevant to medicine must come together in the student's mind. The people and disease SSM helps integration skills to develop. Students study clinical conditions with the help of a mentor, who is a practising doctor. They find and study suitable patients and prepare a dissertation linking basic medical science to real patients' problems.

PHASE 2 – DEVELOPING YOUR SKILLS

The best way to learn clinical medicine is to work with practising doctors. In phase 2, long clinical attachments in hospital and community maximise the opprtunities to learn. In the community, students work as part of the primary care team. In hospitals they are attached to a series of teaching partnerships, groups of two or three clinicians from different specialties, teaching together, whose clinical background and work ensure a wide range of experience. The aim is to develop general skills rather than train in individual specialties. Clearly stated objectives guide learning. Students collate a 'portfolio' of written patient studies throughout to make sure that they cover all the objectives.

The Elective

For one block in phase 2 students devise and undertake a medical project in a setting of their choice. The elective can be anywhere in the world, subject to suitable arrangements. Over 80% of electives are spent abroad.

Preparing for the House Officer Year

After final professional examinations, students shadow the job they will take during the foundation programme in August. They also broaden your experience with a choice of attachments.

Following Your Interests – Intercalating a Year

About 10% of students on the five-year course choose to take an intercalated BSc honours degree, by full-time research. They study for an extra year between years 2 and 3 or 3 and 4, working on a project of their choice, guided by scientists and clinicians who are often world leaders in their field. Some students may enter the MB PhD programme.

Getting to Know One Another

All new medical students on both courses attend a pre-sessional induction week where they are introduced to the Leicester Medical School, the curricula, the educational methods employed and, most important, one another. This helps them both to settle in and to work together with staff as the course progresses.

How to Get a Place

All entrants are selected on the basis of academic performance and personal qualities judged from the application form and at interview. Competition for places is keen. For school-leavers, high grades in appropriate A levels or their equivalent are expected. For the four-year graduate entry course, a first class or good upper second class honours degree in health sciences is required. Some graduates of other subjects are accepted onto the five-year course.

Liverpool L41

A100

SPECIAL FEATURES OF THE COURSE

Problem-Based Learning (PBL) Tutorials

Students are placed in groups of seven or eight with a tutor to discuss a clinical scenario (problem) over a period of two weeks.

Plenary Sessions

Large group plenary sessions in lecture theatres are timetabled, at most, once a day. They are not intended to convey factual information, but are akin to 'keynote addresses', designed to support problem-based learning. They set the scene for a particular topic, highlight important issues and arouse curiosity in relevant areas.

Human Anatomy Resource Centre (HARC)

This resource has recently been developed to provide anatomy-teaching facilities, which are at the cutting edge. HARC is proving to be a national and international model of best practice and many medical schools in the UK are moving towards creation of a similar resource.

Clinical Skills Resource Centre

In much the same way, a Clinical Skills Resource Centre has been built which allows students in their first year to develop their skills on realistic models and sometimes on fellow students. Computer-based learning materials are also available for the acquisition of some skills.

Early Clinical Contact

From second year, the clinical skills learned in the resource centre are applied and augmented in the clinical settings of hospital and general practice. Progressively more days of the week are taken up with clinical attachments as students move through the course. In the final year, all the teaching time is within clinical placements.

Clinical Sciences Resource Centre

The emphasis here is to provide integrated resources to support self-directed learning on the PBL course. These include a computer laboratory with multimedia workstations and copies of recommended course textbooks and research articles.

Communications Skills Course

This comprises fortnightly tutorials which focus on communicating in a doctor/patient relationship.

Clinical Elective Period

All students undertake a five-week clinical elective at the end of their third year, in which they explore a branch of medicine in greater depth. Most use this opportunity to study outside the UK in order to discover how medicine is practised in another country and to experience a different social, cultural and physical environment.

Fifth Year Clinical Apprenticeship

The final year is spent gaining clinical experience in hospitals and the community.

Pre-Registration House Officer (PRHO) Shadowing

Interviews for PRHO posts take place towards the end of year 4. As a result, in the fifth year, students shadow the person who is already undertaking the PRHO post they will eventually take over in the sixth year.

Foundation Year 1 (FY1) Shadowing

In the fifth year, there is an opportunity to shadow a person who is already undertaking an FYI post.

Student Involvement

Student representatives are involved at all levels of planning and delivery of the Curriculum. Each year of the course has a Student Parliament, whose members are responsible for keeping the rest of the student body informed about the work of the faculty and for providing direct input into the management of the programme.

Special Study Modules (SSMs)

Each student undertakes six SSMs during the course, spread across the first four years. These are complementary to the core of the medical course and are intended to broaden experience. They are designed to provide opportunities to explore particular interests, while developing in-depth intellectual and practical skills essential for rigorous scientific and medical practice. Students choose their own SSM to develop individual personal and professional interests. SSMs cover a wide range of topics, including basic medical science, clinical science, behavioural science, epidemiology, and history of medicine, ethics and pathology.

An Intercalated Degree

Students particularly interested in a topic related to medicine, who want to explore this in greater depth than is offered in the SSMs, may choose to take a year out of the medical course (at the end of the fourth year) to undertake an intercalated degree. There is a wide range of subjects available for study in this manner resulting in the award of a BSc, MSc or MPhil degree qualification.

Virtual Resource Centre

The Virtual Resource Centre carries the computer-based resources for the Faculty of Medicine and comprises a series of web pages, which include an electronic version of all student study guides. In addition, it offers web access to an extensive range of medical and scientific learning resources, together with details of all core modules and other resource centres.

Clinical Selectives

In the fifth year, students select two eight-week options drawn from a list of available attachments, enabling them to develop personal interests and provide valuable insight into specialties when making career decisions.

Opportunities for Studying Abroad

The Medical School is closely involved with the Socrates/Erasmus programme, established by the European Union, which enables students to spend part of their study time in another European medical school.

The programme allows students to study within the participating exchange medical school during the fifth year of the course for a period of 16 weeks. As a rule, the exchanges take place during the clinical selective period.

Why Use PBL?

Traditional lecture-based courses have been criticised for encouraging students to gain knowledge in a passive way without understanding how it is applied in clinical practice.

PBL heightens understanding by linking basic medical science with clinical practice very early in the course so that students' interest is stimulated and maintained.

PBL Develops Lifelong Learning Skills

In order to keep pace with the rapid rate of change in science and medicine, doctors need to update their knowledge continually and know how to apply it to patient care. The skills that medical undergraduates gain through PBL will help them to continue learning and applying their knowledge throughout their careers.

Structure of a Typical Two-Week PBL Module

Students are assigned into groups of seven or eight. The group and their tutor meet at the beginning of the first week to consider the clinical scenario, the 'problem', on which the module is based.

The group explores the problem by bringing their prior knowledge to bear and by asking questions. In these ways, students identify areas and topics about which they need to know more.

Students leave the tutorial with their unanswered questions (learning objectives), which each student in the group will use as a framework for further research and study.

Students achieve their learning objectives by using a variety of learning resources, including plenaries (lectures) – maximum one per day, The Human Anatomy Resource Centre, the Clinical Sciences Resource Centre and expert human resources, eg academic and clinical staff.

Checking Progress

The group meets halfway through the module to discuss what has been learned so far. Students have the opportunity to raise any surprises or problems they may have encountered. New learning objectives may emerge. Further independent study follows.

Reflection on the Problem

The group meets again at the end of the module and the problem is reviewed in the light of what has been learned.

The Role of the PBL Tutor

The tutor is not expected formally to teach during the PBL tutorial, but to challenge students' concepts and conclusions, and to ensure that each member of the group is helping the group to progress. The tutor is the key to fostering an open working climate and a successful use of the students' time.

Manchester M20

A106

What does the programme cover?

The aim of the undergraduate medical programme is to produce doctors who are equipped to practise into the second quarter of the 21st century. The emphasis is on self-education, development of critical faculties and communication skills. From the beginning of the programme, students centre on patient problems, using a problem-based learning approach. There are three strands within the curriculum: doctor and society; body and disease; people, health and illness, which require the study of human life at all levels from the molecular to the social. Early experience of clinical and community placements is provided from year 1. Throughout the programme, there are opportunities to pursue individual topics in greater depth.

The first two years of the course consist of four, 12-week semesters, each with an overarching theme: life cycle; cardio respiratory fitness; abilities and disabilities; nutrition and metabolism.

Students are presented with a series of clinically- and/or health-related problems. They are in the form of lecture demonstrations, videos and 'case notes'. Students and staff meet in groups to identify questions raised by the presentation and to define study goals. They will be encouraged to make use of the available resources (such as library and laboratory facilities, histological and anatomical images, specimens and models, as well as the specialist expertise of the staff) to gather information and develop their understanding of the underlying science. Within the group, notes are compared, issues and questions discussed and conclusions drawn.

A variety of lectures will provide you with an overview of a subject, present difficult concepts from an alternative perspective and expand on areas of interest. The intake of students in each year is large (about 360+), but much of the time is spent in smaller groups and there is personal contact with tutors throughout.

From year 3 onwards, students are assigned to one of four major teaching hospitals. Community placements include one day a week in year 3 and an eight-week block in year 5. All of the teaching hospitals have a dedicated skills laboratory, used to allow students to practise various clinical techniques.

Years 3 to 5 build on what students have already learned about human structure, function and behaviour. In year 3, as well as a major skills programme, there are modules on heart, lungs and blood; nutrition, metabolism and excretion. Year 4 builds on year 3, and major themes include mind and movement and family and children. There is also a project option in which students work one-to-one, usually with clinical staff. In year 5 there are five blocks: an elective (which may be overseas), a community placement, two blocks attached to a district hospital (putting clinical knowledge into practice) and a consolidation module (preparing to be a pre-registration house officer).

What are the aims and objectives of this programme?

The aims of the undergraduate medical programme are to enable students to:

- acquire an understanding of health, illness and disease that is firmly rooted in the services underlying medicine;

- acquire clinical skills as a basis for competence;
- develop an insight into patients' needs;
- be capable of monitoring their own performance and learn from others throughout their professional life;
- become aware of ethical issues;
- gain experience in community and hospital settings;
- enter the pre-registration house officer year well-prepared and capable of self-development.

The objectives of the undergraduate medical programme are to ensure that students have acquired and demonstrated knowledge of:

- the range of care problems presented to doctors, their diagnosis, prevention and treatment;
- disease in terms of mental and physical processes;
- factors influencing variability of disease presentation and patient perception of disease.

The programme provides skills encompassing clinical method, including the ability to:

- obtain and record a comprehensive history, perform a complete examination and use the findings to assess patient problems and formulate management plans;
- interpret basic imaging and laboratory-derived data;
- communicate with and inform others about disease process, management and progress, including the breaking of bad news;
- initiate appropriate treatment;
- acquire basic clinical skills, including life support.

It fosters attitudes essential to the practice of medicine, including:

- respect for patients and colleagues that encompasses, without prejudice, diversity of background, opportunity, language, culture and way of life
- respect of patients' rights, particularly in regard to confidentiality and informed consent
- awareness of the ethical responsibilities involved in patient care
- awareness of the need to ensure provision of the highest possible quality of patient care
- the ability to identify personal own strengths and preferences as a basis for making appropriate career choices
- the competence needed to practise medicine as a pre-registration house officer.

Intercalated Degrees

A range of BSc (Hons) can be taken after completion of year 2 or year 4, including physiology, medical biochemistry, pharmacology, physiology/pharmacology/oncology/pathology, anatomy, biomedical sciences or history of medicine. In addition, a Masters in Population Health Evidence is available to students who have completed year 4.

Community Orientation

The programme emphasises community orientation and students have many opportunities to learn how to look after people outside the teaching hospitals, through a one-day-a-week placement in years 2 and 4 and an eight-week placement in year 5.

Clinical Skills

Doctors need skills in communication, history taking, examination and carrying out procedures. Clinical skills laboratories in each of the teaching hospitals help

students develop these skills before putting them into practice.

Student Selected Components (SSCs)

A great deal of emphasis is placed on providing a choice of study outside the core part of the programme. During years 1 and 2, there are opportunities to undertake small projects designed to help students develop their planning, writing and presentation skills. In years 3 and 4, there are two periods each year, in which students can choose to gain further in-depth experience of some aspect of medicine (like anaesthetics, ophthalmology, community paediatrics).

Research

Research is the key to advancing healthcare. Students need to understand how to interpret research studies and how to set about designing and executing their own. In year 4, working closely with a supervisor, they can undertake an 11-week project option research study. The findings of these studies have frequently led to presentation at national and international meetings and to published papers.

Elective

There is an elective period of eight weeks offering the opportunity to study medicine in a different country.

How will you spend your study time?

The first two years are based mainly in the Medical School. In the third year, students are based at one of the major teaching hospitals to gain clinical skills and experience. There are teams of people in these hospitals to provide the experience needed. The fourth year builds on and extends the skills learned in year 3, so that by the final year of the programme, students begin to feel ready to embark on a professional career. To assist in the transition from student to doctor, there is wide experience available in teaching hospitals working alongside the junior doctors.

During years 3 to 5, following on from the problem-based approach in the first two years, there is little didactic teaching, but instead, small group work, which addresses problems specially chosen to illustrate basic principles and disease processes. All common conditions are covered.

Students are assigned to one of the four major teaching hospitals and visit a number of district general hospitals for shorter periods. Each week of the third and fourth-years of the course, students will spend one day in general practice.

Each of the teaching hospitals has a dedicated skills laboratory, which is used to allow students to practise various techniques.

Teaching is based around multidisciplinary teams and will not be subject-specific. The core courses last for 14 weeks in years 3 and 4, and after each, there is a three/four-week SSC, which allows students a degree of choice and specialisation. Since community-based teaching is integrated into the module, one of the four SSCs takes place in the community.

In year 4, the project option offers the opportunity to research one of up to 500 options for up to 11weeks. A written report is submitted and findings are presented. Alternatively, two SSCs may be undertaken.

Year 5 is progression from student to pre-registration house officer. It will involve a series of placements, including district general hospitals, where one or two students are attached to particular consultants to shadow the pre-registration house officer. During this time, you will acquire skills in decision-making and will be expected to defend your decisions rigorously with evidence.

Application and Selection Process

Stage 1 of the selection process is to select those students who fulfil the minimum academic requirements of Manchester Medical School. At stage 2, the UCAS application is read in detail by the admissions tutors and independently by the admissions co-ordinator. Particular attention is given to the personal statement and to the reference from the school/college. The purpose of this assessment is to choose which candidates should progress to stage 3, which is the interview.

Newcastle N21

A106

This degree provides a general medical education. The programme consists of two phases. Phase I lasts for two years, when students study topics in basic and medical science disciplines, with clinical relevance emphasized throughout. These cover normal and abnormal structure, function and behaviour. Modules include:

- cardiovascular, respiratory and renal medicine;
- life cycle;
- nutrition, metabolism and endocrinology;
- thought, senses and movement;
- clinical sciences and investigative medicine;
- personal and professional development;
- medicine in the community;
- student-selected choice.

It's as important to be able to relate well to patients and colleagues as it is to have the basic knowledge. Phase I extends over two academic years and is divided into two stages. During this phase, students learn about normal and abnormal structure, function and behaviour. Contributions come from a variety of basic and behavioural medical science disciplines, with clinical relevance demonstrated through examples of clinical cases. There is also input from other professions allied to medicine, such as nursing, and from the social care and voluntary sectors. People as patients are the emphasis and students come into contact with patients from the very beginning through a link with a GP. Other patient contact includes an attachment to a family for the family study project in stage 1, and an in-depth study of a patient with a chronic illness, the patient study, in stage 2. The patient study is the first opportunity to carry out an in-depth study on a chosen subject. Hospital and general practice visits also introduce students to individual patients, as well as hospital and primary care routines. This introduces the development of the communication skills which underpin history taking. The personal and professional development strand in phase I provides an introduction to ethical reasoning, methods of enquiry and clinical reasoning. At the beginning of the third year, clinical training (phase II), which lasts for three years, starts. For the first year of clinical training, students are allocated to one of our four regional base-units. Clinical teaching takes place in NHS facilities and students may be required to spend prolonged periods at sites away from the university. During phase II, students undertake:

- a 15-week foundation to clinical practice course - introducing basic history taking and examination skills;
- junior rotations – providing clinical experience of specialties like child health, obstetrics and gynaecology, and infectious diseases;
- a 12-week course in clinical sciences and investigative medicine;
- three seven-week options covering clinical and non-clinical medicine – chosen either from a range of topics offered at Newcastle (such as neurosurgery, medical law and paramedic attachments) or in an area of special interest arranged by the individual student;
- a nine week elective – offering the opportunity to study any aspect of medicine, almost anywhere in the world;
- senior rotations in the final year – full-time clinical attachments in areas such as child health, critical care and mental health.

At the end of phase II, students take a short pre-registration house officer 'shadowing' course. This eases the transition to becoming a pre-registration house officer.

An elective?

It's important that students gain as broad an experience as possible. This is why they can spend 11 weeks (including a fortnight's holiday!) studying medicine outside Newcastle University as part of phase II. Recent students have worked in:

- the Paediatric Department at Kilimanjaro Medical Centre in Tanzania;
- the Accident and Emergency Department at University Hospital in Malaysia;
- Community Medicine at Chieng Yun Hospital in Thailand;
- the Department of Medicine Santa Lucia in the Carribean;
- Paediatric Emergency Medicine at the Royal Children's Hospital in Brisbane, Australia.

What skills will I develop?

Newcastle develops the skills students are going to need as professionals. Core skills, knowledge and the right attitude are necessary to be a successful doctor, so students gain experience in:

- clinical and practical skills – a central part of the curriculum;
- communication – both written and spoken;
- teamwork – working with others to complete a task;
- computer literacy and information handling – through projects and assignments;
- reasoning, judgement and decision making – through case discussions, practicals and other assignments;
- self-study techniques – important for postgraduate study and medical learning.

Taught both in formal settings and small group interactions students are given the chance to build on their strengths, tackle weaknesses and develop skills invaluable throughout a medical career.

IS THIS THE RIGHT COURSE FOR ME?

Could you help a child involved in a road accident?

Medicine combines academic theory with a practical application. To help a child involved in a road accident it's necessary to:

- know when to apply the right knowledge;
- have the flexibility to transfer ideas to different situations;
- be able to manage your time and control stress.

Could you find out what was wrong with a patient just by talking to them?

- Are you interested in people and their welfare?
- Can you get on well with them and make them feel at ease?
- Can you express yourself easily and coherently?

Do you enjoy working in a team?

Doctors operate as part of a team with many other people. It's important to communicate well with all these people and work with them towards a shared goal. You could be working with:

- other doctors and consultants;
- nurses;
- radiographers, physiotherapists and other specialists;
- administrative staff.

Oxford O33

A100

WHY STUDY MEDICINE?

Medicine offers a broad range of careers, from general practice to the specialties of hospital practice and medical research. Medicine is an applied science, but it is equally about dealing sympathetically and effectively with individuals, whether they are patients or colleagues. Medicine increasingly poses difficult ethical dilemmas, and, above all, medicine is constantly and rapidly developing and providing a stimulating challenge to practitioners and medical scientists alike.

throughout life, as well as learning about the sciences that underlie modern medicine. These two things – academic skills and scientific knowledge – underpin development as a clinician. Students gain the habits and skills for lifelong self-directed learning, the ability to challenge established practice and develop healthcare based on evidence and a fundamental understanding of health and disease, all of which enable them to respond to changes in knowledge and clinical practice.

WHAT DOES THIS COURSE OFFER?

The skills needed to become a good doctor

To be a good doctor, a sound education and a good medical training are necessary. The Oxford medicine degree develops a range of key skills of benefit

LEARNING TAKES MANY FORMS

Tutorials

The tutorial is the characteristic learning environment in Oxford and provides an important addition to the more standard lectures and practical classes. It forms the focus for independent study each week and provides the chance to discuss ideas and be challenged to think clearly.

On the wards

During the clinical stages, students become an integral part of the clinical team: they clerk patients on the wards, follow them from admission to discharge and present patients to the rest of the clinical team. Students may be required to present a review of the medical literature relevant to patients' illnesses, which will therefore necessitate an understanding of both the patients' clinical management and the relevant clinical research. During most of the clinical course, students are assigned academic tutors who provide bedside teaching. Small-group teaching supplements this tutorial support.

In the community

Community-based teaching is an important part of the clinical course. Early contact in year 4 (year 1 of the clinical course) builds on students' experiences in years 1 and 2 (pre-clinical training) and wherever possible links to hospital-based teaching. Committed and trained GP tutors teach and assess students in year 5 and the school also offers optional attachments in the final year.

Learning independently

In addition to practical classes, tutorials and clinical attachments, students are expected to direct their own learning, identifying weaknesses and actively pursuing areas of interest. To support learning and research, there is access to a network of facilities within the university, colleges and hospitals, including libraries, laboratories, computing facilities and a language centre.

Students can access the school's teaching software and electronic databases of medical and related literature from computers in colleges, university departments, hospitals and general practices; this enables students to keep up to date with the current research, including the latest data on the best treatments for particular disorders.

Teaching is by university, NHS and college staff, including clinicians, research scientists and other healthcare professionals. Most teachers are actively involved in basic or clinical research, which promotes an exciting and stimulating atmosphere for learning. Teachers keep abreast of modern educational practices by attending specialist courses.

PRE-CLINICAL STUDY: COMMENTS OF A STUDENT

Having come from an inner-London comprehensive school, I found Oxford to be a very big change from what I was used to. I found the admissions procedure very fair, but challenging and stimulating at the same time. There was no prejudice to background or schooling whatsoever, and I knew that Oxford would be the place where I would want to spend the next six years of my life.

Studying medicine at Oxford has really increased my passion for the subject. I find the course very rewarding and fascinating. There is a good mix of lectures and practicals that certainly keep you busy. The tutorial system allows me to consolidate the information I learn at lectures and discuss the work with experts in the field at a personal level. The workload is substantial, but I still have time to do things outside medicine. Living in college allows me to meet people studying different subjects. Also, through my involvement with university societies, I have ended up mixing with a wide variety of people from a range of backgrounds and I think all this has enhanced and enriched my experience of university. After all, being a doctor is more than just making the correct diagnosis: it's also about interacting with real people.

Hussein Al-Mossawi

Queen's University Belfast Q50

A100

PERSONAL SKILLS/QUALITIES NEEDED

Motivation/Commitment

When examining the UCAS application, Queen's is looking for evidence of motivation and commitment: work experience – showing an insight into medicine as a career.

Candidates are expected to show that they have made some effort to research the role of a doctor and possible career opportunities available within medicine. It is accepted that direct work experience is not always possible and applicants could choose a combination of the following options.

- Workshadowing (medicine or related discipline)
- Attending medical careers conferences
- Undertaking voluntary work in a care setting
- Talking to doctors or current medical students

Communication skills

Good communication skills are essential and evidence will be sought in both the candidate's personal statement and the referee's reports.

Referee's report

Weight is given to comments on academic ability and predicted grades. Comments on suitability for a career in medicine and the ability to communicate and work well with others are also important.

Health check

All students admitted will be required at the time of registration to provide evidence that they have been successfully vaccinated against hepatitis B or shown to be non-infectious.

INTERVIEWS

Interviews are not held as a matter of course because of the danger of subjectivity and the university leaving itself open to litigious action. Only a small proportion of school-leavers are interviewed, usually because there are queries about certain aspects of their applications. Mature and graduate candidates are routinely interviewed. Applicants are interviewed to assess their motivation, understanding of medicine, communication skills, previous experience and achievements and understanding of the personal and financial consequences of undertaking an undergraduate course in medicine.

THE SUBJECT

The degree course in medicine leads to a qualification that is registrable with the General Medical Council and allows the graduate to practise medicine in its various specialities.

COURSE CONTENT

The Premedical Year

A maximum of five places are available on the premedical year, which is intended for students with science subjects from more broadly-based qualifications than A levels, eg Scottish Highers or Irish Leaving Certificate. Students attend first-year courses in chemistry, physics and biological science. Students must satisfy the requirements of these courses to proceed to the medical course.

The Medical Course

This course, which extends over five years, is integrated, systems-based and student-centred. The scientific background to medicine is therefore taught alongside clinical medicine and, for each system of the body, the whole range of teaching will take place rather than being divided into separate sections, eg anatomy, physiology.

The emphasis is on learning rather than teaching, with less formal teaching and fewer lectures. There is strong emphasis on clinical skills. Students receive teaching in hospitals from as early as the second semester of first year and the fourth and final years are entirely clinical.

Apart from the subjects of the core curriculum, Student Selected Components provide students with the opportunity to select topics from a range available for in-depth study. This includes the opportunity to undertake an elective attachment outside Northern Ireland. At the end of the second or third year, students may also apply to take a year out of their medical course to study for an intercalated BSc degree.

Sheffield S18

A106

Medicine is the study of diseases affecting people. Its scope is vast, encompassing the causes, the nature and the treatment of disease. The school has an international reputation for excellence in its teaching and research and staff who are both expert in their field of practice and in innovative teaching methods. The medical courses at Sheffield offer a broad, clinically-based and extensive education and training leading to the professional qualification of Bachelor of Medicine and Bachelor of Surgery.

The course is based on a patient-centred approach and is designed around common and important clinical conditions. It uses an integrated learning and teaching approach that relates clinical medicine to the underlying medical sciences. Students have the opportunity to develop clinical competencies from the very start.

Teaching includes clinical teaching on wards in hospitals, in clinics both in general practice and hospitals, lectures, seminars, tutorials, small group work, dissection, and personal development supported by experienced tutors and personal mentors. This helps ensure students will be well prepared to work in the National Health Service.

GRADUATE OPINION

'Four months of my pre-registration house officer year have passed already and it's hard to remember what I've done so far! The job is busy and sometimes extremely stressful, but incredibly rewarding at the same time. The learning curve accelerates steeply when you start working. Your confidence and experience build rapidly as you begin to use all the knowledge you have stored in the back of your mind at medical school. The hospitals in Sheffield, and South Yorkshire as a whole, are lively and bustling places to work. It has been really nice to make firm friendships with colleagues in both medicine and the allied professions at work. Nobody could ever prepare you fully for this job before you start, but Sheffield Medical School gave me a firm foundation to embark upon my future career.'

Helena Teige

Graduated June 2003, PRHO Sheffield Kidney Institute

Southampton S27

A100

COURSE FEATURES

General course features are:

- Integrated systems-based programmes in years 1 and 2
- Early patient contact from year 1 in the Medicine in Practice programme
- Study in depth in year 4 to research a topic of the students' choice
- Final year clinical attachments throughout the south of England
- Opportunities to work in an interprofessional team

Placement opportunities

Clinical contact is provided throughout the programme, from year 1. Attachments in regional centres and general practices are available throughout year 5.

Study abroad opportunities

Many students arrange to go abroad for the eight-week elective period in year 4.

Accreditations

Award of the BM degree results in provisional registration with the General Medical Council (GMC). Completion of satisfactory service in hospital and community appointments approved by the university is then required before full registration.

Non-academic criteria

In addition to academic entry requirements the selectors will look at the UCAS personal statement and reference for confirmation of the non-academic criteria and applicants should include this when writing their application. Applicants are asked to demonstrate that they:

- are self-motivated and have initiative;
- are literate and articulate;
- are able to interact successfully with others;
- have learnt from their experiences of interacting with people in health or social care settings. (This may draw on what they have learnt from their own experience, such as friends or family or some formal activity, like paid or voluntary work, or work shadowing.)

Interviews

School-leaver applicants are not normally interviewed and the absence of an interview should not be interpreted negatively. Selected international applicants and the majority of selected mature applicants are interviewed as part of the selection process. Each interview is conducted by two members of staff and would normally include a member of the selection committee.

Offers

All offers are conditional upon achieving or providing evidence of qualifications that meet the academic entry requirements. In addition, as applicants must be able to fulfil the duties of a doctor as outlined by the GMC in their document *Good Medical Practice*, both the offer and continued registration on the course are conditional upon completion of satisfactory health screening, which is assessed in confidence by staff in the Occupational Health Department.

Disability

Applicants must be able to fulfil the duties of a doctor as stated by the GMC in their document *Good Medical Practice*.

St Andrews S36

A100

THE COURSE OVERVIEW

The medical course at St Andrews has a long-established reputation as providing an excellent scientific basis for clinical training.

- At the heart of the course is a series of patient-centred workshops designed to demonstrate the application of scientific knowledge to common medical conditions. Patients provide the context within which students develop relevant clinical and communication skills, together with appropriate professional attitudes.

- The first year of the curriculum is the pre-honours component of the degree programme. It lays the foundations for medical training by providing an overview of the organisation of the body and an initial examination of the molecular and physiological basis of metabolism, genetics and disease. Students study aspects of medical history, philosophy and ethics to provide a background for understanding the concepts of professionalism and responsibility in medicine. A series of family attachments and interviews provide insights into health psychology.

- The second and third years comprise the honours component of the degree programme. Patient workshops continue to provide the clinical focus for skills training and the detailed study of normal and abnormal structure and function in all the body systems. These themes incorporate the relevant aspects of public health and health psychology.

- In the second year, students also attend a scheme in which a wide range of healthcare professionals design and deliver 10 individual community programmes. As well as receiving teaching in a classroom environment, students have the opportunity to shadow healthcare professionals working in the community.

- The final elements of the honours programme consist of two components, a major student-selected component that will take the form of an honours-level project and the applied medicine module. This module will draw together major topics and provide an excellent opportunity to apply your knowledge and skills to novel clinical problems.

FIRST YEAR

To introduce students to a career in medicine, St Andrews explains what is meant by the term 'medical profession' and what that means for a doctor in training. Medical education not only involves a scientific understanding of health and disease, but also how to communicate and work with patients and colleagues, how to develop professional thinking and problem-solving skills, and how to find and interpret information.

The first year consists of two modules, **foundations of medicine 1 and 2**. The central theme of the entire curriculum is a series of patient workshops that illustrate the importance of the medical science topics students will be tackling. Small group work provides the opportunity to work in teams and develop a clearer understanding of the science. Clinical skills that relate to specific patients are introduced throughout the course.

In **foundations of medicine 1**, the basic molecular and cellular processes that underpin our understanding of metabolism and genetics will be studied alongside the basic organisation of the body from cells and tissues to organ systems.

In **foundations of medicine 2**, the study of cell behaviours and interactions will be extended to provide an understanding of the function of the musculo-skeletal system. St Andrews offers the opportunity to observe human structure directly by dissection of the entire body during your three-year course. A three-dimensional understanding of the body and its organisation is the essential basis of clinical examination and imaging. Medicine is considered to be an art as well as a science. Clinical cases and scenarios are used to stimulate discussion of the moral and philosophical issues leading to an understanding of medical ethics.

The **Honours** programme comprises a series of modules that build upon the knowledge base established in foundations of medicine 1 and 2. The normal and abnormal structure and function of each of the body systems (eg respiratory, gastrointestinal and renal) are studied in depth and this includes the scientific basis of disease mechanisms in each of the body systems. Patient workshops again underpin this integrated approach and provide a strong clinical emphasis.

During the honours years, students develop a deeper understanding of the practice of medicine through the use of literary works and video presentations that

MANCHESTER MEDICAL SCHOOL

enhance critical thinking, reflective practice and decision-making.

The final semester has a strong emphasis on independent learning. Students have an opportunity to conduct a research or library project, or special study module to pursue an area of their own interest at an advanced level. In the same semester, the applied medicine module is completed. This course is designed to enhance professional thinking skills, integrate major topics and provide opportunities to consolidate clinical skills and patient examination techniques.

- St Andrews' graduates and third year students from the University of Manchester combine to begin their clinical training together.

- The University of Manchester has the largest medical school in Europe with outstanding clinical facilities.

- Students find that the St Andrews' medicine course integrates very successfully with the excellent clinical training they receive at Manchester Medical School.

Clinical training is based at one of four teaching hospitals. The same core curriculum is delivered at each using common clinical cases chosen to illustrate basic principles and disease processes.

The teaching approach is largely problem-based throughout. In the spring of the second year at St Andrews, students are given the opportunity to visit all four hospitals. The Medical School can usually accommodate preferences.

- The first clinical year consists of a major clinical skills review and modules on 'heart, lungs and blood' and 'nutrition, metabolism and excretion' and also special study modules.

- The second year builds on and extends the skills learned in the previous year, and the major themes of 'mind and movement' and 'family and children'. There is also the opportunity to pursue a research option, where students work one-to-one, usually with clinical staff.

- The third year supports the progression from medical student to house officer and aims to help students apply their knowledge and sharpen their skills. It involves shadowing house officers at different general hospitals. One of the eight-week modules is an elective in which students follow any approved medically-based subject. Many students choose to study overseas, where they can broaden their experience and investigate other forms of health service delivery and a different spectrum of illness.

Bristol B78

Medicine Graduate entry (4 years)
Four-year full-time degree – A101

ABOUT THE COURSE

- The four-year (fast-track) MBChB programme offers additional education and professional training for graduates in medical sciences or other para-medical professions. A degree in medicine equips students for a professional career as a doctor. The programme has a strong emphasis on integrated teaching, early clinical experience, a strong science base and extensive tutorial group support.

- The transitional first year of the course builds on existing knowledge of the medical sciences and their relevance to clinical medicine, introducing concepts relating to the human basis of medicine. On successful completion of the first year, students continue with the full final three years of the medical programme.

SPECIAL FEATURES

- Initial medical teaching primarily takes place in the School of Medical Sciences in the main university precinct and in NHS Trust hospitals and general practices in the city.

- During years 2 to 4, teaching takes place at a clinical academy – for half of the year at an academy in Bristol and the other half at a 'regional' academy. Students are given placements at as many of the different academies as possible to widen their experience and engage fully in clinical activities across the region, training alongside other healthcare professionals.

- The programme's strength is research-informed teaching. All departments are internationally renowned for their research, so teaching is by people who are world experts in their fields. Research strengths include neuroscience, cancer biology and immunology.

- The programme includes a series of student-centred projects, known as 'student-selected components', which provide the opportunity to study particular areas of interest in more depth, as well as the opportunity to study modern languages.

COURSE OPTIONS

Students on this fast-track course will follow the same teaching schedule as the five-year A106 students, but are exempt from the 'molecular and cellular basis of medicine' unit, and complete the remainder of the year 1 and 2 units in one year instead of two. Certain students may be exempt from the anatomy component of the programme; this will depend on their previous qualifications.

- The programme is divided into a series of compulsory units with associated assessments. Most units are further sub-divided into elements (subject areas). Running throughout the programme are five themes – communication skills, evidence-based medicine, ethics and law, disability and rehabilitation, and whole person care – that cross year boundaries and provide continuity for essential themes that permeate all medical practice. Students study their own interests through the student-selected components (student-centred projects).

- The first year provides formal teaching on the body systems and their diseases, in which medical science and clinical departments collaborate. The second year involves full-time clinical attachments in combined medicine and surgery, musculoskeletal medicine, and mental health.

- The third and fourth years continue clinical training, covering more specialist areas and, in the final year, preparing for qualification.

Leicester L34

A101

LAYING THE FOUNDATIONS

Students develop the knowledge, skills and attitudes necessary to communicate with patients, examine them, and interpret their observations. They take a core course, plus special study modules (SSMs) where they choose topics to suit their interests and aspirations. Phase 1 is modular, over three semesters, including 18 core modules and two SSMs, in recognition of graduates' prior learning.

CLINICAL SKILLS

Much of the time in phase 1 is spent in direct clinical work, meeting patients very early on. Clinical and communication skills are developed in a structured way, first by attachment to a family, working with volunteers and actors simulating patients, and then by work with real patients in hospital.

MEDICAL SCIENCES

Medical sciences are taught through integrated, interdisciplinary modules. Applied subjects like pathology, microbiology and pharmacology are introduced very early, so that students can immediately understand both normal and abnormal function.

Social and Behavioural Medicine

Patients have social and psychological dimensions to their lives that affect the kind of illnesses that they suffer from and how they react to them. Many modules emphasise these aspects so students can appreciate the behavioural and social dimensions in clinical practice.

LEARNING HOW TO LEARN

Medicine requires a commitment to lifelong learning. Leicester aims progressively to develop skills of self-directed learning. Learning is largely by group work and by problem solving. There is lots of time for self study.

DEVELOPING SKILLS

The best way to learn clinical medicine is to work with practising doctors. Students spend nearly all their time in phase 2 on long clinical attachments in hospitals and the community. The aim is to develop general skills rather than individual specialties.

THE ELECTIVE

In phase 2, students devise and undertake a medical project in a setting of their choice. The elective can be anywhere in the world, subject to suitable arrangements. Financial assistance may be available. Over 80% of electives are spent abroad.

Liverpool L41

A102

COURSE STRUCTURE

This course differs from the five-year (A100) course in the following ways.

- Students have an extended year 1, starting at the end of August and ending in late July.

- There is early clinical contact from November of year 1.

- Students undertake only three special study modules.

PROBLEM-BASED LEARNING TUTORIALS (PBL)

Students are placed in groups of seven or eight with a tutor to discuss a clinical scenario (problem) over a period of two weeks.

PLENARY SESSIONS

Large group plenary sessions in lecture theatres are timetabled, at most, once a day. They are not intended to convey factual information, but are akin to 'keynote addresses', designed to support problem-based learning. They set the scene for a particular topic, highlight important issues and arouse curiosity in relevant areas.

EARLY CLINICAL CONTACT

From November of year 1, the clinical skills learned in the resource centre are applied and augmented in the clinical settings of hospital and general practice. Progressively more days of the week are taken up with clinical attachments as you move through the course. In the final year, all the teaching time is within clinical placements

CLINICAL SCIENCES RESOURCE CENTRE

The emphasis is to provide integrated resources to support self-directed learning on the PBL (problem-based learning) course. These include a computer laboratory with multimedia workstations and copies of recommended textbooks and research articles.

COMMUNICATIONS SKILLS COURSE

This comprises fortnightly tutorials focusing on communicating in a doctor/patient relationship. Students try out their skills with simulated patients (actors) at the end of the course.

CLINICAL ELECTIVE PERIOD

Students undertake a five-week clinical elective at the end of the second year, in which they explore a branch of medicine in greater depth. Most use this opportunity to study outside the UK to appreciate how medicine is practised in another country and to experience a different social, cultural and physical environment.

Newcastle N21

A101

WHAT DOES THIS COURSE COVER?

This accelerated programme is designed for graduates of any discipline and others with previous professional experience. It allows students to qualify in four years instead of five. The programme is taught in two phases. Phase I of the programme is completed in one extended year as opposed to the two years of the standard programme. Teaching and learning focuses on a case-led approach, of which some elements will be problem-based. The course is organised around seven subject strands:

- cardiovascular, respiratory and renal medicine;
- life cycle;
- nutrition, metabolism and endocrinology;
- thought, senses and movement;
- clinical sciences and investigative medicine;

- medicine in the community;
- personal and professional development.

Given the prior experience of graduate entrants, an element of the eighth strand, student-selected choice, is omitted from phase I of the accelerated programme. Students are organized into small study groups, each allocated a senior medical tutor providing general academic and personal support, as well as facilitating weekly teaching sessions. Clinical training (phase II), which lasts for three years, starts in the second year. Phase II is identical to the five-year programme. Clinical teaching takes place in NHS facilities and students may be required to spend prolonged periods at sites away from the university.

Phase II includes:

- a 15-week foundation to clinical practice course – introducing basic history-taking and examination skills;
- junior rotations – providing clinical experience of specialities, such as child health, obstetrics and gynaecology, and infectious diseases;
- a 12-week course in clinical sciences and investigative medicine;
- three seven-week options covering clinical and non-clinical medicine – chosen either from a range of topics offered, or in a chosen area of special interest;
- a nine-week elective – which is an opportunity to study any aspect of medicine, almost anywhere in the world;
- senior rotations in the final year – full-time clinical attachments in areas such as child health, critical care and mental health.

CAN I SPEND TIME ON AN ELECTIVE?

It's important to gain as broad an experience as possible, so there's the opportunity to spend 11 weeks (including a fortnight's holiday!) studying medicine outside Newcastle University. Students can choose any aspect of the subject and go anywhere in the world.

Oxford O33

A101

THE COURSE FOR YOU?

The four-year course at Oxford is very intensive, and has a very strong basis in academic science (both clinical and laboratory-based). It also assumes that high-calibre graduates will wish to use teaching sessions for advanced study and discussion, and not for didactic teaching of basic core material.

The Oxford four-year course is not for you if you think you will need help to assimilate basic core material. It covers in four years most of the material that is usually covered in Oxford's standard six-year course: this produces a great deal of pressure, and requires not only considerable academic strength, but also very strong self-discipline to cope with the volume of study. It is not for students who are keen to get on to clinical practice with the minimum amount of academic science.

Oxford puts great emphasis on the scientific practice of medicine, because it believes that clinical practice benefits greatly from an understanding of the underlying science. The course may be right for students who are academically strong, interested in the scientific basis of medical practice, and have the self-discipline to plan their studies in such a way as to be able to cover a large and intensive syllabus. Students who fit this description may gain a great deal from Oxford's very strong academic and clinical teaching.

STUDENT PROFILE

I've found the graduate-entry course both interesting and exciting. We've been learning clinical skills right from day one, both on the wards at Milton Keynes and in primary care at Aylesbury. These sessions have been structured around our pre-clinical work, which is seminar-based, rather than a series of lectures. There's plenty going on socially in Oxford – in the city itself, in the colleges, and also events at the medical student club, Osler House.

Nicolas Brown
Graduate Entry Student

Southampton S27

A101

COURSE FEATURES

- Learning in the first two years is designed around a series of clinical topics.
- Substantial clinical experience is gained in the first two years based in Winchester.
- Graduate groups form a focus for learning.
- Common learning with the five-year programme exists in some lectures and practicals in years 1 and 2, and in clinical attachments in the third and fourth years.
- Final-year attachments are dispersed around Southampton and house officer shadowing follows final exam.

PLACEMENT OPPORTUNITIES

- Substantial clinical experience is gained from year 1, with attachments in first two years based at Winchester. There are attachments in regional centres and general practices throughout year 4.

STUDY ABROAD OPPORTUNITIES

- Possibilities exist for an attachment abroad for a four-week module in year 4.

ACCREDITATIONS

- Award of the BM degree results in provisional registration with the General Medical Council (GMC). Completion of satisfactory service in hospital and community appointments approved by the university is then required before full registration.

Bristol B78

A104

- This six-year course is designed for students whose entry qualifications are not suitable for direct entry to the five-year MBChB course. It offers a pre-programme preliminary year, where students take year 1 units in chemistry, physics and anatomical science. On successful completion of the preliminary year, you will join the regular five-year MBChB programme.

- A degree in medicine equips students for a professional career as a doctor. The programme has a strong emphasis on integrated teaching, early clinical experience, and a strong science base, with extensive tutorial group support.

- The programme is divided into three phases. Phase 1 provides patient contact straightaway and teaches the general principles underlying behavioural science and basic medical science (two terms). Phase 2 comprises formal teaching on the body systems with full-time clinical attachments in year 3 (two years); phase 3 is clinical training, covering more specialist areas (two years).

SPECIAL FEATURES

- Initially, medical teaching primarily takes place in the School of Medical Sciences, which offers excellent facilities and is situated in the main university precinct. You will also be taught in the numerous NHS Trust hospitals and general practices in the city.

- During years 3 to 5, students attend a clinical academy – for half of the year, they are in an academy in Bristol and for the other half, they are based at a 'regional' academy. Across the three clinical years, students are placed at as many academies as possible in order to widen their experience. This helps students engage fully in ongoing clinical activities across the region, training alongside other healthcare professionals.

- Bristol views its strength as being in research-informed teaching.

- At the end of year 2, or exceptionally year 3, students may be able to intercalate an extra year in order to study for an honours BSc degree.

- The programme includes a series of student-centred projects, known as 'student-selected components', in which students study particular areas of interest in more depth.

- There is also the option to spend time studying abroad (elective study) for two months in the final year. In addition, the Bristol Medical School was a pioneer in the European Credit Transfer Scheme, and students can spend three to six months at a participating European medical school in year 3, and receive credit for academic work successfully undertaken there.

Cardiff C15

Medicine (foundation course)
Six-year full-time degree – A104

WHY SHOULD I STUDY MEDICINE (FOUNDATION COURSE) AT CARDIFF UNIVERSITY?

The integrated curriculum blends basic medical sciences and clinical disciplines within a structure that combines traditional learning methods with a problem-centred approach. During the course, there are three strands of learning and training: knowledge and understanding; skills and competencies; and attitude and conduct. The third strand is the key feature of professional development and it is expected that students demonstrate these attributes from an early stage.

COURSE INFORMATION

The foundation programme is designed for students who have demonstrated high academic potential, but who do not meet the specific subject requirements for entry to the five-year medical programme, ie those who have non-science subjects or a combination including no more than one of biology, chemistry and physics.

Students on the one-year modular programme study 12 modules alongside students of other science disciplines. Normally, modules include biological and chemical sciences or other subjects, such as mathematics. Modules are available in other subjects, like psychology and languages. The combination of subjects is selected according to the students' prior qualifications

The first phase of the programme introduces all the major systems of the body and the cellular and tissue processes, including their operation in the normal and diseased states. Additionally, early clinical experience fosters an appreciation of the person as an individual and the role of healthcare in society. During this stage, students undertake an extended case study of the development of a baby born to a local family. Other clinical and non-clinical special study component (SSC) projects in these early years include diverse opportunities to follow areas of personal interest.

The clinical experiences in year 2 are short attachments to local hospitals and with GPs and the completion of a course in basic life support. In year 3, this part of the course continues with the foundation clinical skills course, manual handling skills and a period gaining nursing experience. Tutors in the Clinical Skills Laboratory help students to acquire, practise and refine skills in a supportive environment. Similarly, the initial acquisition of communication skills is principally through sessions with tutors and surrogate patients.

By the fourth year, the practical aspects of communicating with patients and clinical skills develop through a series of clinical attachments in primary care and in hospitals. Initially, clinical experience centres on the more commonly encountered diseases and issues in surgical care, and this is supported by the linkage to the pathological basis of the disease processes and the pharmacological strategies.

The later clinical modules extend into speciality practice and patient management, eg acquiring the special skills of managing the care of children, the elderly or the mentally ill. Other areas of medicine require different examination skills. To acquire these skills, it is important that the clinical training is accompanied by the continuum of medical science, and that these experiences are gained in a wide variety of settings. Therefore, students spend periods attached to clinical teams in hospitals and community healthcare settings throughout Wales, with periods of consolidation and review of progress in Cardiff.

In the final year, knowledge and skills are extended through attachments covering serious and acute illness, including intensive care and trauma, and community medicine. This period consolidates clinical and communication skills, as well as providing experience of general practices, both urban and rural, and hospices. In addition, students complete a course in advanced life support.

A substantial proportion of the final year is devoted to SSCs: the elective period, which is a long-standing feature of the medical course in Cardiff, and the senior clinical project. The elective is an opportunity to study any subject of interest at medical centres, research units or community practices around the world ensure students have a friendly reception as well as interesting and challenging experiences. In contrast, for the senior clinical project, students choose any clinical aspect of the course for an in-depth study.

Finally, immediately before qualifying, a period of clinical consolidation in the hospital where students will be working as doctors prepares them for the role of a house officer and smoothes the transition into being a junior doctor.

Dundee D65

A104

- Students have the opportunity to study medicine in a fully integrated medical school and hospital with extensive teaching and research facilities, which serve both teaching and clinical needs.

- The course is problem-orientated, student-centred and community-based in a medical school highly renowned for leadership and innovation. The 12 Dundee learning outcomes, now adopted by all Scottish medical schools, direct learning and assessment throughout the course. The focus of learning is approximately 100 core clinical problems.

- Students obtain real clinical experience from year 1 with direct patient contact.

- There is a choice of what to study from a wide range of SSC modules (Student Selected Components) and students can even propose their own to reflect particular interests. SSC modules form one third of the course.

- Students can also choose from a range of clinical attachments in Dundee, Tayside and elsewhere in Scotland and the UK. In the final year, they have the opportunity to travel anywhere in the world to undertake a period of elective study.

- Students are part of a caring community providing healthcare for Tayside, Fife and further afield, and have access to a wide range of school facilities, including lecture theatres, teaching laboratories, library, integrated self-teaching area, computer suite and Clinical Skills Centre.

Manchester M20

A104

WHAT DOES THE PROGRAMME COVER?

The aim of the undergraduate medical programme (MBChB) is to produce doctors who are equipped to practise into the second quarter of the 21st century. The emphasis is on self-education, development of critical faculties and communication skills. From the beginning of the programme, students centre on patient problems, using a problem-based learning approach. There are three strands within the curriculum: doctor and society; body and disease; people, health and illness, which require the study of human life at all levels from the molecular to the social. Early experience of clinical and community placements is provided from year 1. Throughout the programme, opportunities are provided to pursue topics of individual interest in greater depth.

The first two years of the MBChB consists of four 12-week semesters each with an overarching theme:

- life cycle;
- cardio respiratory fitness;
- abilities and disabilities;
- nutrition and metabolism.

Students are presented with a series of clinically- and/or health-related problems in the form of lecture demonstrations, videos and 'case notes'. They meet in groups with other students and staff to identify questions raised by the presentation and to define study goals. They make use of the available resources (such as library and laboratory facilities, histological and anatomical images, specimens and models, as well as the specialist expertise of the staff) to gather information and develop an understanding of the underlying science. Members of the group compare notes, discuss issues and questions, and draw conclusions.

There is an opportunity to attend a variety of lectures. Some provide an overview of a subject; others present difficult concepts from an alternative perspective; others expand on areas of interest. The intake of students in each year is large (about 360+) but a lot of time is spent in smaller groups and students remain in personal contact with tutors throughout their studies.

From year 3 onwards, students are assigned to one of four major teaching hospitals and visit a number of district general hospitals for shorter periods. Community placements include one day a week in year 3 and an eight-week block in year 5. All of the teaching hospitals have a dedicated skills laboratory, which is used to practise various clinical techniques.

Years 3 to 5 build on students' knowledge of human structure, function and behaviour. In year 3, as well as a major skills programme, there are modules on heart, lungs and blood; nutrition, metabolism and excretion. Year 4 builds on and extends year 3, and major themes include mind and movement and family and children. A project option offers the chance to work one-to-one, usually with clinical staff. In year 5, there are five blocks: an elective (which may be overseas), a community placement, two blocks attached to a district hospital (putting clinical knowledge into practice) and a consolidation module (in preparation for being a pre-registration house officer).

Sheffield S18

A104

The pre-medical science foundation course gives students with a non-scientific background the necessary basic scientific knowledge to undertake the medical course. The course prepares students for entry to phase 1 of the medical course and is based at the Loxley Centre of the Sheffield College. During the course, students visit local hospitals to see the clinical relevance of the science they are studying. Entry requirements are good grades (AAB or better) in arts subjects at A level or a non-science degree.

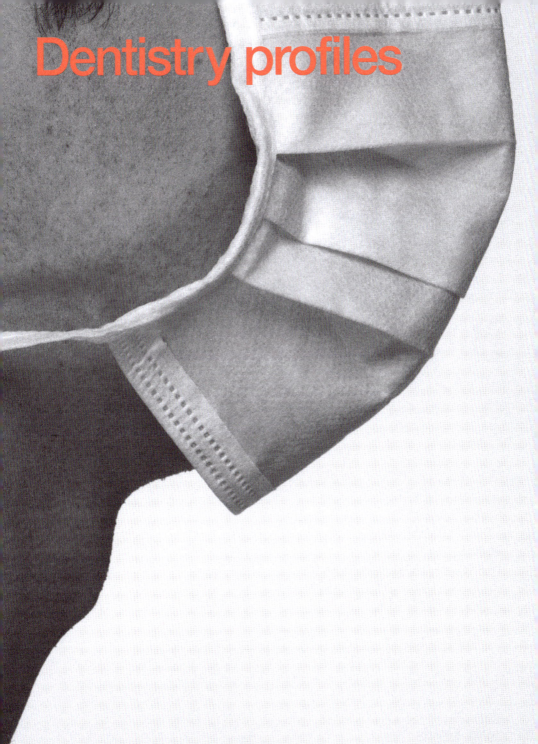

Dentistry profiles

Birmingham B32

A200

DESIRABLE SKILLS/QUALITIES AT ENTRY

Dental work experience

It is essential that all candidates should have some experience of working in a dental surgery.
The majority of time should have been spent with a general dental practitioner, with sessions spent observing specialists if possible.

Communications skills

Although dentistry is academically and technically demanding, gaining patient confidence is also essential in the delivery of care. Clear, positive and informed communication contributes greatly to patient co-operation. Therefore it is necessary to demonstrate this ability in discussion with staff at interview.

Liking people

Today's dentist works as part of a team, which includes not only the patient, but also a hygienist, technician and nurse. It is important therefore that applicants can relate well to people. Empathy and a desire to benefit society are important aspects of a dentist's professional life.

Teamwork

Dentistry is a team effort and the dental surgeon leads the team in every way, from support and guidance, to the hiring and firing of staff. The team's effectiveness determines the success of the practice. Though such responsibilities can be onerous, these skills will be developed through the course. This aspect of work should be viewed as an opportunity, rather than a disadvantage.

Practical skills

Dentistry is not only academically demanding, but also technically exacting. Some indication of practical ability is important for prospective dental students. This is often in the form of musical ability or art (drawing, painting, sculpture etc), needlework, model making, or anything that shows the ability of hand-to-eye co-ordination.

SKILLS DEVELOPED ON THE COURSE

Prescriptive and diagnostic skills

On completion of the course, students should be capable of independent dental practice: to diagnose, prescribe and carry out a course of treatment to render a patient dentally fit. However, at present, all registered national health dentists also carry out one year's post-graduation training known as 'vocational training'. During this time, students work with a vocational trainer who provides support and advice. The vocational training period is salaried and on satisfactory completion, the trainee can seek independent positions in practice.

Practical skills

The level of practical skills will be developed to the point where fine and detailed work can be carried out with confidence and accuracy in a difficult environment.

Interpersonal skills

One of the most important aspects of a successful dental practice is interpersonal skills. These will be developed through training in written and oral communication and providing an insight and understanding of patients' fears and needs.

Leadership skills

Leadership skills are developed throughout the course by dealing with other members of the support team. Students learn to work with nurses, develop referral techniques to hygienists and prescriptive skills to dental technicians. These skills will eventually enable them to guide and support their own team.

IT skills

IT is an essential part of modern practice and throughout the course these skills are refined and developed so that informed judgements can be made about requirements.

Research and analytical skills

Throughout the course, students are required to analyse and appraise published material for content and value. This skill is enhanced during an elective period when students' research is written and refereed to provide understanding and appreciation of such work.

Bristol B78

Dentistry – first BDS (pre-dental) entry
Six-year full-time degree – A204

ABOUT THE COURSE

- A dental surgeon is primarily concerned with oral health and the prevention of dental disease, but must also have a wide appreciation of general medicine. Dentistry is an intellectually stimulating career, largely based on scientific principles, but also requiring artistic flair.

- This six-year course is designed for students whose entry qualifications are not suitable for direct entry to the five-year BDS course.

- It offers a pre-programme foundation year, where students take year one units in chemistry, physics, and anatomical science. Even though these units are provided by the Faculties of Science and Medical and Veterinary Sciences, students are regarded as 'dental' students.

- On successful completion of the foundation year, students join the regular five-year BDS programme. Throughout the programme, there is an emphasis on the prevention of disease and whole patient care.

- The second and third years of the course are pre-clinical, and are spent in the Medical School, but with regular opportunities to gain clinical experience in the Dental Hospital. Clinical training takes over in the final three years.

- At the end of the third year, students have the opportunity to intercalate a year in the Faculty of Science or the Faculty of Medical and Veterinary Sciences, studying for a BSc honours degree in one of the subjects of the pre-clinical curriculum. On completion, they rejoin the dental programme.

- The Dental School has long-established dental and cultural links with Hannover Dental School and each year an exchange programme takes place.

- At the end of the fifth year, there is an elective study period, when students undertake a short dentally-related project at an approved academic institution anywhere in the world. Limited financial assistance is available.

- The BDS programme is divided into 17 units, each of which covers a particular subject that is taught and assessed as a whole. Each unit may be subdivided into two or more elements for teaching purposes.

Bristol B78

Dentistry – second BDS entry
Five-year full-time degree – A206

ABOUT THE COURSE

- A dental surgeon is primarily concerned with oral health and the prevention of dental disease, but must also have a wide appreciation of general medicine. Dentistry is an intellectually stimulating career, largely based on scientific principles, but also requiring artistic flair.

- The five year programme at Bristol has been carefully structured and is designed to ensure a stimulating university education leading to the degree of Bachelor of Dental Surgery. Throughout the programme, there is an emphasis on the prevention of disease and whole patient care.

- The first two years of the course are pre-clinical, and are spent in the Medical School, which gives students the chance to sample life as a typical student before the clinical training takes over in the final three years. However, from the first year there are regular opportunities to gain clinical experience in the Dental Hospital.

COURSE OPTIONS

- The BDS programme is divided into 17 units, each of which covers a particular subject that is taught and assessed as a whole. Each unit may be subdivided into two or more elements for teaching purposes, with internal assessments contributing in various ways.

- During the first pre-clinical year in the School of Medical Sciences, a thorough understanding of the basic medical sciences is gained. However, students will be able to appreciate the clinical relevance of these subjects by observing and working alongside senior students on the Dental School clinics. Additionally, a practical unit in applied dental materials provides an opportunity to develop manual dexterity and to gain a better understanding of the anatomy of the tooth and of the techniques seen in the clinics.

- In the second pre-clinical year, the programme broadens to encompass behavioural science, molecular pathology and microbiology, pharmacology, and an in-depth study of oral tissues in health. Special study elements give students the opportunity to study a modern language or sign language, or to conduct a research project.

- Social dentistry is taught throughout the BDS programme. Students are introduced to psychology and sociology, and become familiar with subjects like law and ethics, and dental public health.

- In year 3, a broad study of human disease is undertaken (this is known as medicine and surgery elsewhere). It includes visits to other hospitals and clinics. In the following two years, oral diseases are studied in depth.

- Clinical dental practice is undertaken throughout years 3, 4 and 5. Following the completion of the element of basic dental restorative techniques, students take responsibility for treating patients within the clinical departments, under the close supervision of members of staff.

- Years 4 and 5 include residences and rotation at the Bristol Royal Infirmary in Accident and Emergency and other wards.

SKILLS DEVELOPED ON THE COURSE

Subject-Specific Skills

Students gain the knowledge and skills needed to become a professional dentist and will be able to practise in the UK as well as in many other countries.

General Skills

As well as professional skills, students also develop other interpersonal and technical skills required as a dentist. Here are some examples.

- Initiative and independence of thought.

- Skill in written and spoken communication.

- Excellent IT skills.

- The ability to work as part of a team.

- The ability to take responsibility for both patients and team members.

- A continuing commitment to education throughout their career and they will be able to undertake independent study, as changing techniques and new materials present new challenges.

Cardiff C15

A204

COURSE INFORMATION

The aims of the dental programmes of study are to teach students dentistry in a training environment appropriate to their professional aspirations. They enable students to combine knowledge, skills and judgement with an appropriate attitude to deliver a high standard of professional care.

The School of Dentistry has developed an integrated curriculum which is designed to meet the challenge of providing training to work in a rapidly changing educational and clinical environment. Features of the programme include the following.

- Early clinical contact – clinical teaching is introduced at an early stage. Students spend a half day each week during the first year at the School of Dentistry and University Dental Hospital.

- Innovative teaching and learning methods, including the use of computer-assisted learning, video-based teaching and IT tools.

- An integrated curriculum blends the basic dental sciences and the clinical disciplines within a structure that combines traditional learning methods with aspects of a problem-centred approach.

- Opportunities to teach and practise in community clinics, district general hospitals and satellite academic units.

- An emphasis on inter-professional education. Joint teaching sessions are arranged with students of dental hygiene and therapy.

Students spend most of their first year studying with Cardiff School of Biosciences, learning the basics of anatomy, physiology and biochemistry, which underpin dentistry, through a series of lectures, seminars and practicals. They also spend one afternoon per week at the University Dental Hospital observing clinics, learning about clinical procedures, professionalism, dental terminology and the role and responsibilities of the dental team.

Following successful completion of the first year, students continue with the foundation topics integrating with modules covering oral ecosystems, which embrace the biology and biochemistry elements of dentistry. These themes are enhanced and supported by modules on human diseases, through which students learn aspects of medicine, pharmacology and surgery required by the dentist. In addition to these lectures, seminars and practicals, students are introduced to clinical dentistry. They examine themes of dentistry in the wider community, behavioural science and ethics, as well as continuing the family study programme started in the first year.

The third and fourth years develop themes incorporating clinical dentistry, human diseases and dentistry in the wider community, covering topics such as integrated restorative care, prosthodontics, periodonotology, paediatric dentistry, orthodontics, statistics, oral surgery, medicine and pathology and dental public health. The amount of time spent in the clinics treating patients and developing interpersonal and clinical skills also increases.

The final year is spent mainly in the community. Students spend their time in general dental hospitals, local and outreach clinics, secondments and Erasmus.

The underlying philosophy of the clinical teaching in the School of Dentistry has always been one of total patient care and this principle means that students are personally responsible for the oral and dental health of the patient in a similar way to what they will experience after qualification.

Cardiff C15

A200

WHY SHOULD I STUDY DENTISTRY AT CARDIFF UNIVERSITY?

The School of Dentistry is committed to, and renowned for, excellence in teaching and research. With its outstanding facilities and friendly atmosphere, it attracts students worldwide. The school is large, successful and has long-standing experience of providing professionally recognised dental teaching, research and patient care.

COURSE INFORMATION

The aim of the dental programme is to teach students to practise dentistry in a training environment appropriate to their professional aspirations. This enables them to combine and use knowledge, skills and judgement, developing an attitude appropriate to the delivery of a high standard of professional care.

The School of Dentistry has developed an integrated curriculum designed to meet the challenge of providing training appropriate to a rapidly changing educational and clinical environment. Students need to have both the flexibility and attitude to adapt to the working environment. Features of the programme include the following.

- Early clinical contact – clinical teaching is introduced at an early stage. Students spend a half day each week during the first year at the School of Dentistry and University Dental Hospital.

- Innovative teaching and learning methods, including the use of computer-assisted learning, video-based teaching and IT tools.

- An integrated curriculum that blends the basic dental sciences and the clinical disciplines within a structure that combines traditional learning methods with aspects of a problem-centred approach.

- Opportunities to teach and practise in community clinics, district general hospitals and satellite academic units.

- An emphasis on inter-professional education. Joint teaching sessions are arranged with students of dental hygiene and therapy.

The first year provides the basics of anatomy, physiology and biochemistry, which underpin dentistry, through a series of lectures, seminars and practicals. One afternoon per week will be spent at the University Dental Hospital observing clinics, learning about clinical procedures, professionalism, dental terminology, and the role and responsibilities of the dental team.

Following successful completion of the first year, students continue with the foundation topics integrating with modules covering oral ecosystems, which embrace the biology and biochemistry elements of dentistry. These themes are enhanced and supported by modules on human diseases, through which students learn aspects of medicine, pharmacology and surgery required by the dentist. In addition to these lectures, seminars and practicals, students are introduced to clinical dentistry. They examine themes of dentistry in the wider community, behavioural science and ethics, as well as continuing the family study programme started in the first year.

The third and fourth years develop themes incorporating clinical dentistry, human diseases and dentistry in the wider community, covering topics such as integrated restorative care, prosthodontics, periodonotology, paediatric dentistry, orthodontics, statistics, oral surgery, medicine and pathology and dental public health. The amount of time spent in the clinics treating patients and developing interpersonal and clinical skills also increases.

The final year is spent mainly in the community. Students spend their time in general dental hospitals, local and outreach clinics, secondments and Erasmus.

The underlying philosophy of the clinical teaching in the School of Dentistry has always been one of total patient care and this principle means that students are personally responsible for the oral and dental health of the patient in a similar way to what they will experience after qualification.

Dundee D65

A200

WHY STUDY DENTISTRY AT DUNDEE

A dentist's task is to ensure that patients have healthy teeth and mouths, thus contributing to their general health and wellbeing. This involves not only treating dental and oral diseases, but also helping to prevent them. This needs to be done in a patient, tactful and considerate manner, recognising the needs, reactions and fears of patients. Becoming a dentist necessitates a high degree of technical skill, accurate clinical judgement, intelligence and a logical, inquiring mind. Dentists also need to be fit, healthy and have a cheerful and kindly disposition.

The school provides modern clinical, lecturing, tutorial facilities for the dental education of a student intake of 55 to 60 each year. The hospital and school building is in the main university precinct, only a short distance from the library, the students' union and the university sports centre. It has its own lecturing, tutorial, laboratory and clinical facilities. These include a combined self-teaching centre with audiovisual aids and a dedicated computer-aided learning suite, along with reference material. Closed-circuit television is used in appropriate cases.

The school has a very good record of attracting selected students to an intercalated **Bachelor of Medical Science (Honours)** degree course, taken usually in the year following year 2. The subjects available for study for the BMSc (Hons) are:

- anatomy;
- biochemistry;
- cellular and molecular basis of disease;
- forensic medicine;

- medical psychology;
- physiology.

TEACHING AND ASSESSMENT

Teaching methods used involve a mixture of techniques, including lectures, tutorials and seminars, and practical laboratory and clinical teaching. Assessment methods for both class and degree examinations vary, with, for example, essay papers, practicals and multiple-choice questions. The school has recently introduced objective clinical testing in the form of objective structured clinical examinations and structured clinical objective testing. Viva voce (oral) examinations are also employed as appropriate.

A full course outline is available via the Dundee entry profiles on www.ucas.com

Dundee D65

A204

A dentist's task is to ensure that patients have healthy teeth and mouths, thus contributing to their general health and wellbeing. This involves not only treating dental and oral disease, but also helping to prevent them. This needs to be done in a patient, tactful and considerate manner, recognising the needs, reactions and fears of patients. Becoming a dentist necessitates a high degree of technical skill, accurate clinical judgement, intelligence and a logical, inquiring mind. Dentists also need to be fit, healthy and have a cheerful and kindly disposition.

The school provides modern clinical, lecturing, tutorial facilities for the dental education of a student intake of 55 to 60 each year. The hospital and school building is in the main university precinct, only a short distance from the library, the students' union and the university sports centre. It has its own lecturing, tutorial, laboratory and clinical facilities. These include a combined self-teaching centre with audiovisual aids and a dedicated computer-aided learning suite, along with reference material. Closed-circuit television is used in appropriate cases.

The predental year introduces:

- molecular sciences;
- evolution and biodiversity;
- environmental biology;
- biomolecular mechanisms;
- genes, heredity and development.

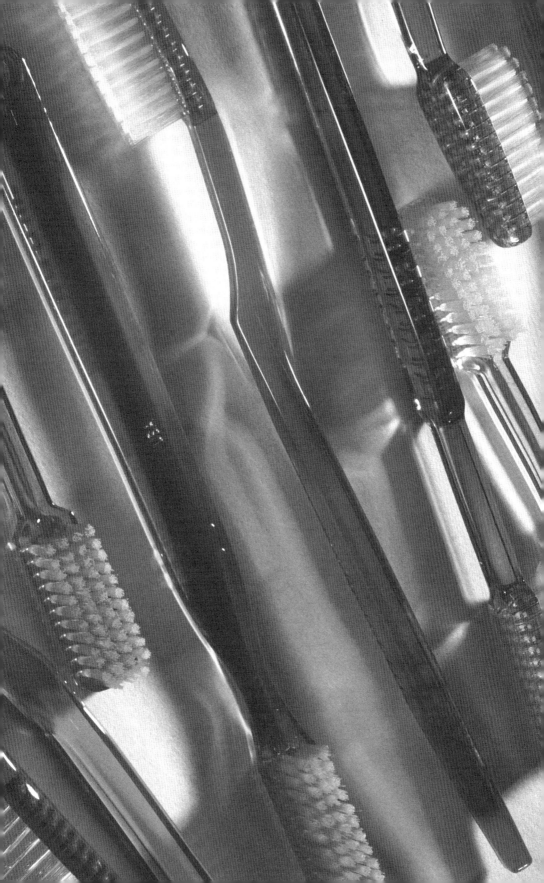

Glasgow G28

Five-year full-time degree – A200

Work shadowing

As well as the usual academic entry requirements, it is essential that all applicants have work-shadowing experience, preferably within a general dental practice setting. Applicants with less than three days' (or equivalent) work-shadowing experience will not be invited to interview. The three-day requirement does not necessarily mean that all contact time must be with the dentist. It should include time with the dentist, but it is equally important to understand the roles of other members of the dental team.

It is preferable that you provide evidence of an interest in dentistry and that you also have an understanding of the career you are choosing and what it means to be in the profession.

Activities within school and outside of school

Applicants must have participated in some form of extra curricular activity within the school, and outside of school. These activities should demonstrate that you:

- are able to analyse information and be capable of independent thought;
- are able to be self-critical and self-motivating;
- are able to plan and think on the spot and enjoy problem solving;
- are capable of working in a team and also have the capacity to act as a leader;
- have a caring, empathetic nature;
- are trustworthy and respectful of the views of others;

- Can put people at ease, demonstrating good interpersonal skills;
- Have evidence of manual dexterity, creativity and spatial awareness.

Portfolio

All applicants are required to submit a portfolio as part of the admissions process. Applicants who do not submit a portfolio will not be invited for interview.

Career prospects

Most dental graduates become general dental practitioners. Other possible careers lie in the hospital service, the community dental service, in the universities and in the armed forces. In all spheres of dentistry, education is recognised as a lifelong experience and continuing education is increasingly recognised as important for the professional development of a graduate.

If you choose to follow a career in National Health Service general dental practice, you will be required to undertake a period of vocational training designed to ease the transition between dental school and general dental practice. This vocational training period lasts one year. However, in some parts of the country, it has been voluntarily extended to a two-year period of general professional training, to provide experience in the provision of dental care in both primary and secondary settings.

You may choose to study for one of the higher diplomas or degrees awarded by the Royal Colleges or the universities. The University of Glasgow offers various postgraduate degrees: PhD, DDS, MSc. This would be essential if you chose to follow a hospital or university career, but appropriate further qualifications may be pursued by those in all branches of the profession.

Contact with the Dental School can be maintained during your professional life through the Glasgow Dental Alumnus Association, founded in 1979. One of its first achievements was the establishment of the Glasgow Dental Educational Trust and the creation of the West of Scotland Postgraduate Dental Centre, the only one of its kind in the UK. In premises adjacent to the Dental School, the centre includes a 10-chair clinical unit and has helped Glasgow remain at the forefront of postgraduate training in dentistry. The centre also houses a Distance Learning Unit with up-to-date computer technology in which continuing education programmes are being developed for general dental practitioners to use in their own surgeries.

King's College London (University of London) K60

Five-year full-time degree – A205

THE DENTISTRY DEGREE

The programme incorporates the latest thinking in dental education – early clinical exposure, an emphasis on ideas as well as facts, integrated teaching of all subjects, with an emphasis on a systems approach, and a dimension of choice of special subjects by the student. The integrated nature of the programme means that basic science teaching will relate to clinical practice and clinical teaching will be underpinned by scientific understanding. You will have contact with patients from the first few weeks of the first year and will be encouraged to assume an appropriate level of responsibility for patient care at an early stage. The programme emphasises whole patient care, which implies consideration of the patients' total dental and medical needs, rather than just the provision of items of treatment. Most of the teaching is carried out in small groups where students and staff get to know each other well.

THE PROGRAMME

The programme has three main components. The first consists of subjects common to medicine and dentistry, progressing from biomedical sciences, through behavioural sciences, epidemiology, pathology and microbiology to human disease. The second includes oral and dental aspects of the biological sciences leading to an understanding of the diagnosis, prevention and treatment of oral and dental diseases and disorders and the effects of systemic disease on the oral and dental tissues. The third component consists of the clinical and technical aspects of dentistry with the provision of comprehensive oral and dental healthcare for patients of all ages.

These components are vertically integrated with a larger proportion of basic sciences at first and a larger clinical component at the end. Throughout the five years of the programme, you will, in addition to acquiring the practical skills necessary to become a dentist, acquire communication skills, personal management skills, information technology skills and an appreciation and analysis of ethical and legal issues in dentistry.

Examinations are held at the end of each year, and a percentage of the marks for each examination are derived from in-course assessment, which may take the form of essays, practical tests or project work.

INTERCALATED BSc

At the end of year three, you will have the opportunity to take an intercalated BSc degree, which allows you to pursue the subjects of your choice in greater depth. The advantage of studying at a multifaculty institution such as King's College is that units can be taken in a wide variety of subjects. For example, you may wish to study clinically-relevant subjects and related topics, such as health services management or psychology, as well as more traditional subjects, such as neuroscience and biochemistry. You may even seek to further your language skills.

Leeds L23

A200

YEAR 1

Laying the foundations

- Five-week 'induction course'– the induction course introduces ways of learning to be a dental student and a dentist. It covers oral health, what can go wrong and how to approach helping to put it right – helping students to find out what dentistry is really all about.

- Classes will provide a firm foundation for students to understand and assess scientific methods and principles.

- Clinical sessions in the Dental Institute and outreach clinics provide early experience of clinical dentistry.

- Variety in learning and teaching – self-directed, group work and working with other oral health students are all part of the Leeds approach.

- Courses in year 1: induction, the mouth and clinical practice, health and health promotion, disease, defence and repair 1, pain and anxiety, personal and professional development 1.

- The dental team – experience will be gained of working with dental nurses, hygienists and therapists in outreach clinics and in the institute.

YEAR 2

Building experience and knowledge

- Classes provide an integrated study of nutrition and its impact on oral health and disease.

- Clinical experience provides experience in some simple, well-defined areas of clinical skills and practice.

- The dental team – experience will be gained of working with dental nurses, hygienists and therapists in outreach clinics and in the institute.

- Personal and professional development continues to expand learning power and an understanding of the student's role as a developing professional.

- Courses in year 2: nutrition and metabolism, disease, defence and repair 2, clinical skills and related clinical practice, personal and professional development 2.

YEAR 3

A pivotal year

- Classes cover the study of wellbeing and illness and place renewed emphasis on professional and communication skills directly relevant to patient care.

- Clinical experience sees students working more closely with patients, as well as studying clinical skills and dentistry in more depth.

- An in-depth research project is undertaken to improve students' ability to acquire and evaluate knowledge independently.

- The dental team – students analyse the roles of members of the dental team, as well as writing simple prescriptions for dental hygienists, therapists and dental technicians.

- Courses in year 3: wellbeing and illness, communication, clinical skills and related clinical practice, research project, personal and professional development 3.

At the end of year 3:

- an honours degree in oral health sciences will be awarded to students who have completed successfully the requirements to this level of the programme, but decide not to continue the programme of study.

YEAR 4

Amassing experience

- Classes take students through the study of mastication, sedation and aspects of human disease relevant to dental care.

- Clinical experience further develops understanding and skills and spans the specialist areas of restorative dentistry, paediatric dentistry, oral surgery, oral medicine, oral pathology, oral radiology and orthodontics.

- Optional courses provide an opportunity to widen the knowledge base of students to include subjects like psychology or a foreign language.

- Courses in year 4: human disease, child-centred dentistry, complex adult dentistry and clinical practice, anxiety and sedation, personal and professional development 4.

YEAR 5

The culmination

- Classes ensure that students develop the attributes, skills and knowledge to make the transition to professional life, as well as deepening their understanding of human disease, ageing and its impact on oral care.

- Clinical experience continues, providing a sound basis for continuing professional development.

- Shared learning focuses on working with and managing members of a dental team.

- Optional courses are currently being formulated to offer the opportunity to study subjects like advanced restorative dentistry, advanced child-centred dentistry and business management, to participate in the Socrates European exchange programme or to undertake a second research project.

- Courses in year 5: integrated clinical practice, ageing, preparing for the world of work, personal and professional development 5.

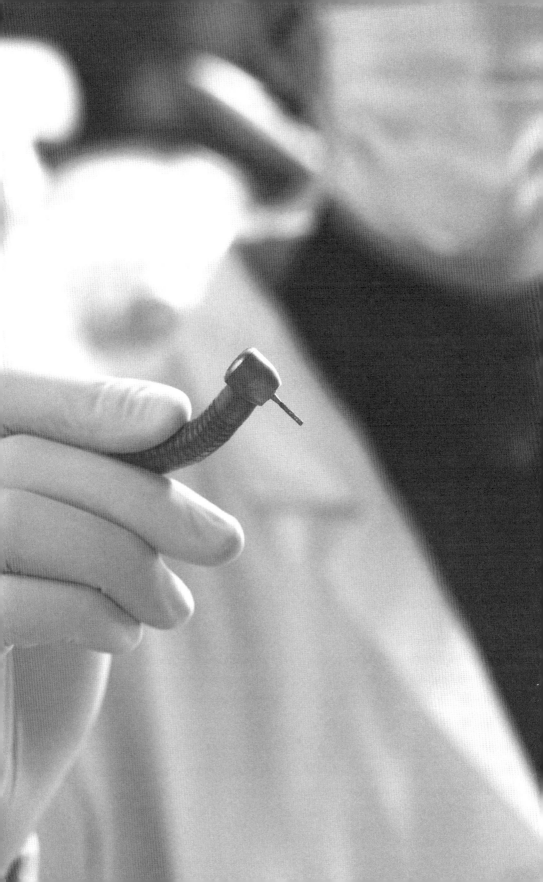

Liverpool L41

Five-year full-time degree – A200

Dr Lawrence Mair, Head of Division of Clinical Dental Sciences, says that, "Besides being highly skilled surgeons, dentists are increasingly becoming leaders of small teams of professionals that include dental hygienists, dental therapists, dental technicians and dental nurses. The aspiring dentist needs to be strongly motivated towards healthcare, with good interpersonal and organisational skills. Dentistry is constantly developing and the programme at Liverpool provides not only the training for practice on graduation, but it also equips the students for continual professional development throughout their career."

PROGRAMME CONTENT

Phase I comprises the first two semesters of the programme and has three basic elements. The first is an introduction to basic medical sciences, where students study via a 'problem-based learning' (PBL) course taken in conjunction with the first year medicine students, and which occupies three days a week, including self-study. The second element is an introduction to operative dental surgery, including practical operative technique, undertaken as a special dental module during the second semester. Finally, an introduction to preventive dentistry includes participation in a communication skills course.

Phase II, which occupies the second, third and fourth years, again has three strands. It is an integrated, modular course planned to cover applied aspects of the basic medical and dental sciences, as well as clinical laboratory sciences with medicine and surgery. It is delivered through a series of clinical scenarios, employing didactic learning methods and training in the practical skills of dentistry through the supervised treatment of patients in the dental hospital, and continuing instruction in preventive dentistry and behavioural sciences. During the fourth year, the medical aspects of dentistry are developed in a course in oral diseases, sedation and general anaesthetics; law and ethics are also introduced, as well as a course in the development and evaluation of new knowledge. This course includes study design and statistics, measurement in dentistry and how to review the literature in a structured way.

All this prepares the student for planning and carrying out their period of elective study towards the end of the fourth year or beginning of the fifth. This compulsory elective study period gives the student time to carry out an independent study. The study may be undertaken within or outside the university; many students travel overseas, for which small bursaries may be available.

Phase III is the final year of study, consolidating theoretical knowledge and clinical experience in preparation for the final examination. A series of seminars, tutorials and discussion sessions are held; these can be multidisciplinary, and the dental students are joined by basic medical scientists and experienced clinical teachers to discuss and evaluate controversial issues and clinical topics.

Intercalated degrees: Students who do well in their phase I examinations have the opportunity to spend a year in one of the Honours Schools of the Faculty of Science studying for the additional degree of BSc (Hons). This option has now been extended to the end of phase II to increase the range of subjects available for intercalated study. More information is available on the university website.

Manchester M20

Dentistry (BDS first-year entry)
Five-year full-time degree – A206
Dentistry (BDS pre-dental-year entry)
Six-year full-time degree – A204

WHAT CAN THE COURSES OFFER ME?

The Manchester dental programme aims to develop professional and ethical dentists who can demonstrate the ability to:

- take a patient-centred approach to clinical care within the dental team;

- apply the skills, knowledge, attributes and abilities to practise safely and efficiently;

- be reflective practitioners, committed to lifelong learning.

WHAT DO THE PROGRAMMES COVER?

The Manchester dental programmes are fully integrated five- and six-year programmes. Clinical subjects are taught alongside the basic dental science subjects. From very early in the programme, students study aspects of clinical dentistry. A key feature of BDS dentistry is the use of enquiry-based learning (EBL). This spectrum of approaches is characterised by student-driven enquiry, including problem-based learning (PBL), small-scale investigations (eg case studies), projects and research activity.

YEARS 1 AND 2

The first two years of the five-year programme focus on the behavioural and biological basis of dentistry. The PBL approach allows the varied subject areas to be covered in an integrated manner. The introduction to practical clinical dentistry begins in the first year with sessions spent practising basic clinical and technical skills. This is followed in the second year by the development of operative skills. Initial learning takes place in the clinical skills areas and on patient simulators. At the same time students are introduced to the materials they will use in future practical work.

YEARS 3 AND 4

The third year provides the knowledge and skills to deliver preventive and clinical dentistry. The breadth and depth of clinical dentistry develops through the programme and student work in outreach clinics, treating both child and adult patients, begins.

YEAR 5

The fifth year of the programme builds on and integrates knowledge and skills gained in previous years, so that students can provide comprehensive patient care and are prepared to begin to practise independently following graduation.

The Manchester dental programme aims to:

- deliver a curriculum that meets the educational requirements of the General Dental Council;

- equip students with the knowledge and skills to pursue a successful career in dentistry;

- successfully deliver the curriculum by employing the appropriate range of teaching, learning and assessment strategies;

- provide appropriate academic staff, laboratory, clinical and other facilities to ensure a high quality learning environment and experience;

- provide the opportunity for teaching, training and learning in outreach clinics to offer experience of dental care in different communities;

- monitor the dental programme to ensure that it is appropriate to the changing needs of the profession;

- provide effective academic and pastoral support;

- instil in students the importance of research.

OBJECTIVES

On successful completion of the programme, students should have the following.

Knowledge and understanding of:

- the scientific information that forms the foundation of dentistry;

- the broad principles of scientific thought, including experimental design;

- the safe and effective care of patients;

- the legal and ethical requirements for the practice of dentistry.

The professional skills to:

- utilise their knowledge to solve problems and engage in independent thought;

- define and formulate questions;

- be able to undertake independent study;

- undertake the dental care of patients in a safe and effective manner;

- recognise clinical limitations and make appropriate referrals;

- work as part of a dental team,

- prepare and present written and verbal reports utilising the appropriate information technology.

SPECIAL FEATURES OF THE PROGRAMME

PBL
PBL in dentistry was pioneered in the UK at the University of Manchester. Students work in groups to plan their own learning in relation to descriptions of clinical cases. This method encourages the development of skills fundamental to dental practice, like communication, team work, independent learning, information retrieval and processing.

Integration
The integration of non-clinical and clinical aspects of the programme ensures the relationship between science subjects and the elimination of disease is immediately apparent. This philosophy allows for the rapid transfer of relevant research findings to the clinics.

Outreach clinics
Emphasis is placed on exposing students to dentistry outside the confines of the dental school through custom-built community clinics. Treatment needs are high, there is no shortage of patients and students gain valuable experience of working as part of a team of dentists, dental nurses, hygienists, therapists and receptionists.

Teamwork
The importance of teamwork is emphasised throughout. The School of Dentistry also provides a BSc programme in oral health sciences. Thus, student dentists and student dental therapists learn side by side, working together to provide patient care, simulating the modern world of dental practice.

Research
There is an emphasis on research throughout. Of particular note is the use of critically appraised topics, in which students pose a clinical question, eg 'Is water fluoridation an effective means of preventing tooth decay?', and assess the existing published literature to draw conclusions. Through the review process, students acquire the skills to assess, in a meaningful way, new developments in dentistry. Student reviews are added to the dental school's database of critically appraised topics and are published on the website.

Intercalated BSc
Outstanding students can take an extra year to study for an intercalated BSc (Hons) degree. This is partly taught and partly research based. The choice of subjects is varied and ranges from pathology to psychology to the history of medicine.

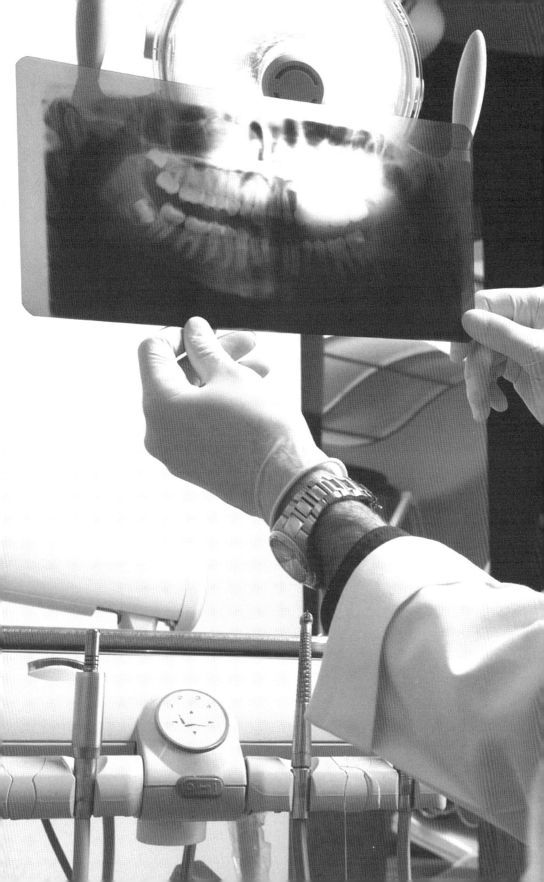

Newcastle N21

A206

WHAT DOES THIS COURSE COVER?

This degree gives you the skills and knowledge needed to become a professional dentist with full responsibility for the oral healthcare of patients. Divided into five integrated stages, the first two (lasting around 18 months) provide a firm grounding in the scientific knowledge needed for later clinical work. Students are introduced to basic and applied biomedical science subjects including:

- molecules, cells and tissue;
- anatomy of the head and neck;
- cardiovascular and respiratory systems;
- nutrition and diet;
- special oral science courses – such as dental tissues and craniofacial development.

Students also 'shadow' a more senior student to see the relevance of their studies to later clinical work.

Stage 3 onwards focuses on clinical training (lasting around three and a half years). From simple filling and root treatments on 'phantom heads' – model heads using natural teeth and clinical materials – students move on to manage patients and give simple treatment under supervision. The emphasis is on the prevention of dental disease as well as its treatment, so students learn how to:

- prevent disease, plan treatment, treat dental decay and place fillings;
- undertake root treatments, treat gum disease and make dentures;
- extract teeth and possibly even undertake simple surgery;
- use radiographs (X-rays), local anaesthetics and deal with cross-infection;
- deal with patients – including the special skills needed to treat children.

Stages 3 and 4 see students continuing to study the theory of dentistry, and developing the complexity and range of their clinical skills. Courses covering many aspects of human disease and their management provide an insight in to how disease affects patient care. Half the time on stage 4 is spent on clinical patient care and almost all of stage 5 is spent in this way. Observing and even treating patients using advanced techniques such as orthodontics, dental implants and intravenous sedation, students also get the chance to see patients receiving specialist treatment, including restorative dentistry, maxillofacial surgery and paediatric dentistry.

CAN I SPEND TIME ON AN ELECTIVE?

Yes. It's important to gain as broad an experience as possible. This is why students can spend time studying dentistry outside the university at the end of stage 4, choosing from:

- abroad – students have been as far as America, China and Australia;
- at a specialist unit in the UK – such as an oral and maxillofacial or trauma unit;
- on a research project in Newcastle – current research varies from year to year.

Electives are optional, so aren't assessed. They last for up to nine weeks – involving the clinical vacation, plus an extra couple of weeks from term time. Many students take the opportunity to help provide community dental services in remote areas or work with a charity medical service. Others observe high tech hospitals in the USA or flying dentist practices in the outback of Australia. As increasing globalization has made experience of another country more important than ever, Newcastle also developed exchange links with Helsinki in Finland, where students can spend three months at the beginning of stage 4 studying topics in dentistry.

WHY CHOOSE NEWCASTLE?

Excellent facilities. Students use some of the best and most up-to-date teaching equipment in the country, with access to:

- a clinical skills laboratory – for pre-clinical practical training;
- a dental hospital – with excellent clinical facilities;
- computer clusters and modern computing facilities;
- regularly updated clinical equipment – so students gain experience with the most modern technology.

High quality teaching. Staff are actively involved in dental research, so teaching is up-to-date. We use a variety of learning methods including:

- lectures and seminars;
- laboratory demonstrations – including closed-circuit TV;
- CAL (computer aided learning);
- practical laboratory work and clinical demonstrations;
- clinical dental practice – students take responsibility for patient treatment.

Emphasis on clinical practice throughout the degree culminates in stage 5 when that accounts for almost all the student's time.

Intercalated degrees. Students often have an area of particular interest and so they are given the chance to study for an additional degree by taking a year out from their dental studies. Intercalation is available for BDS students after completion of stage 2 (into any of the BSc courses in the area of biomedical science, for example, physiological sciences, medical microbiology and immunology), or after stage 4 (into the MRes programme). The degrees are based around a research project and dissertation. The opportunity to work independently during this year broadens experience and helps students make decisions about their future career.

WHAT SKILLS WILL I DEVELOP?

Newcastle emphasizes developing interpersonal as well as technical skills. Employers look for a wide range of different skills, so students gain plenty of experience in:

- tcamwork – working with others to complete a task;
- communication – both written and spoken;
- computer literacy – through projects and assignments;
- management and initiative – taking responsibility for patients and other members of the team;
- self-study techniques – through projects and assignments;
- independent study skills – managing a workload on your own initiative;
- practical ability – students need manual dexterity;
- flexibility – using knowledge in more than one area.

If you think you have all these skills and can balance the different demands, then you'll be able to make a real difference to society!

QMUL Q50

Five-year full-time degree – A200

Being a dentist involves more than just doing fillings and scaling teeth. Dentistry is a major branch of medicine dealing with all aspects of the care of the mouth:

- prevention of dental diseases – caries and gum disease
- repair of the damage caused by these diseases if they aren't actually prevented
- screening for oral cancers – dentists, rather than doctors usually pick up on these
- management of trauma – the results of road accidents, children falling off bikes and skateboards, fights and so on; this can involve both dental and facial repairs
- orthodontics – basically braces (for children and adults; it's never too late to wear a brace!)
- oral surgery – the extraction of unrestorable, unwanted or buried teeth

- 'lumps and bumps' – mouth ulcers, white patches and assorted pains. The mouth is the mirror of the body, so students need a very good understanding of general medicine.

Dentistry graduates have:

- excellent communication skills: no dentist can manage without them
- cognitive skills: or the ability to reason and to interpret information
- IT skills
- team-working ability: there are several group projects
- team-leadership skills
- time-management ability: especially if students undertake an overseas elective, which they plan themselves.

The five-year programme is divided into three stages.

Stage 1: Fundamentals of Dentistry

This part of the course introduces biological principles. Students acquire the study skills needed throughout the course, including working effectively in small groups, researching information and using IT as a learning tool.

Through lectures, seminars, clinical sessions and computer-assisted learning students are given a preview of the entire course and introduced to the key topics addressed at every stage, including:

- the normal biological structure and function of cells
- the body's main organs and systems
- the effects of illness on people and their families
- the impact of environmental and social factors on health
- clinical skills.

Stage 2: Integrated Clinical Studies

Students learn about the various body systems in health and disease, with topic areas geared towards the requirements of a dentist in training. Particular emphasis is placed on oral biology, with the study of the normal structure and function of the oral cavity and adjacent tissues leading on to consideration of abnormalities and diseases of the mouth and related structures.

The effects of systemic disorders on oral health, and the management of dental patients, also form an important part of the study programme. Throughout the course, students develop a wide variety of practical clinical skills through the experience of treating patients. Therefore, a considerable amount of time will be spent in clinical contact with patients, in addition to complementary educational activities, such as seminars, laboratory class work, tutorials, computer-assisted learning, projects and library work.

The courses are delivered in a series of modules, including oral cavity, prosthodontics, human health and disease, child oral health and plaque-related diseases. The modules are presented in an integrated and multidisciplinary way, incorporating input from all relevant disciplines. The dental curriculum aims to achieve a high level of integration between the clinical and basic science components of the course. Selected study modules are included to provide opportunities to study areas of personal interest in greater depth. Subjects such as pathology, pharmacology, social and psychological sciences, medical ethics and law, clinical and communication skills, dental materials science and the prevention of oral disease, run throughout the course.

Stage 3: Preparation for Dental Practice

The final part of the curriculum is an opportunity to consolidate the knowledge, skills and behaviour developed throughout the course in preparation for professional dental practice. At this stage, small groups of six to eight students work together to tackle a problem and consolidate knowledge acquired over the previous four years. Newly-qualified dentists usually have to complete a year of approved vocational training following graduation.

KEY ELEMENTS OF THE COURSE

The course provides a broad knowledge of aspects of medicine and dentistry and their application to the diagnosis, prevention and treatment of oral and dental disease and deformity. The school believes in a team approach to training, and students work alongside trainee dental nurses, therapists and technicians. An holistic approach to dentistry is encouraged. This involves studying the human sciences – sociology and psychology – looking at patients' attitudes to oral healthcare and the dental profession, whilst also learning about the community aspects of dentistry.

Queen's University Belfast Q75

A200

The dental undergraduate programme is five years in duration with the first two years integrated with the medical curriculum. Graduates are awarded the Bachelor of Dental Surgery degree, which is approved by the UK's General Dental Council.

The School of Dentistry is co-sponsored by the UK's National Health Service and Queen's University. This partnership of the National Health Service and the university provides a school in which teaching and clinical service are fully integrated in a combined dental school and dental hospital. The school has a core ethos of high quality patient care in which the clinical service, teaching and research are integrated to ensure excellence in all three areas.

The school has a staffing complement of 180 clinical and clinically-related staff and treats approximately 45,000 patients per year.

THE COURSE

Year 1 provides an introduction. Modules cover cell structure and function, including histology, biochemistry and genetics. A module on science, society and medicine deals with the scientific, information technology, sociological and psychological aspects of medical/dental practice. A family attachment programme commences in this semester and continues throughout years 1 and 2. It provides students with the opportunity to observe the impact of a health problem on family life. Communication skills training also commences in this phase and continues through the undergraduate programme.

In the spring semester, a course commences in which each system in the body is studied in turn, with the emphasis on normal structure and function. Alongside this is an introductory clinical course in which students learn the approach to patients and how to undertake the examination of the different parts of the body. This is taught partly in hospital, partly in general practice and partly in the Clinical Skills Education Centre.

The second year introduces students to clinical dentistry. The course philosophy is of health promotion, and a whole-patient approach to dental care. This introductory course has a number of components which provide an introduction to:

- dental health education;
- core clinical concepts;
- clinical management;
- clinical procedures;
- biomaterials;
- computing;
- project work.

The course introduces students to the behavioural sciences programme, which runs throughout the rest of the clinical course and highlights 'communication skills', 'working in dental practice', and 'working with special needs', eg old persons, AIDS, anxiety.

Year 3 expands on pathology, microbiology and pharmacology and commences the study of medicine and surgery. These subjects occupy morning sessions; in the afternoons, students' introduction to clinical dentistry continues. Medicine and surgery courses introduce human disease as it affects patients in the context of dental practice. There are opportunities to see patients with medical and surgical problems at ward rounds conducted at the Royal Victoria Hospital. At the end of the medicine and surgery courses, three

weeks are spent in full-time attachments to medical and surgical clinics and wards as well as accident and emergency departments.

At the end of the third year, there are opportunities for students to undertake a further year of study in any of the subjects listed below and obtain an Intercalated Honours Bachelor of Science (BSc) or Bachelor of Medical Science (BMedSc) degree.

The main content of **the fourth year** is related to the clinical disciplines under the major headings of dental surgery, conservation, periodontics, prosthetics, orthodontics, paediatric and preventative dentistry.

General anaesthesia and sedation

There will be an introductory course of lectures in general anaesthesia with additional lectures in sedation. Students are allocated to sedation sessions and there will be a two-week full-time clerkship in anaesthetics based at the Department of Anaesthetics.

Behavioural sciences

The behavioural sciences programme runs throughout the undergraduate course. The aim of the course is to increase awareness of the psychological and sociological parameters of health and illness, and to introduce the concept of a psychobiological model of health.

Dissertation

The student dissertation has been structured to incorporate a problem-based element. The aims of the student dissertation are to:

- develop an attitude to learning that is based on curiosity and the exploration of knowledge, rather than its passive acquisition;
- develop clinical thought, an awareness of scientific method and an insight into research methods;

- complement other aspects of problem-based learning within the curriculum.

Elective

A four-week period has been set aside for the fourth year elective period. During this time, all students undertake a period of study/clinical experience in one of the clinical or related disciplines. Students are encouraged to spend this elective period outside Northern Ireland.

In year 5, clinical sessions in oral surgery/oral medicine, conservation, prosthetics, periodontics and paediatric and preventive dentistry will continue. As the year progresses, the course aims to provide opportunities to introduce a number of components which have been designed to:

- complement the clinical training and expertise already gained;
- emphasise the changing patterns of dental disease and healthcare;
- emphasise the concepts of total patient care;
- contribute to the preparation for independent practice.

It is beneficial that a proportion of the time spent in these components could be outside the School of Dentistry.

The objectives are to ensure that the dental graduate is capable of promoting communal effort to broaden the type and amount of dental healthcare for the population, and to widen students' views of the professional opportunities and challenges of dentistry.

Sheffield S18

Five-year full-time degree – A200

This is a five-year course. Content is under continual review to ensure it incorporates the rapid advances taking place in dentistry.

During the first year of the course, students study biochemistry, anatomy, physiology and oral anatomy, largely in classes designed for dental students. In addition they attend an introductory clinical course in the Dental School.

In the second year, teaching begins to concentrate on the clinical dental subjects, studying the common afflictions of teeth and their supporting tissues, the properties of dental materials and how they are used. Extracted teeth set in model heads enable students to learn a wide variety of operative procedures and, under close supervision, to begin treating patients.

As students gain experience, they learn more complex and specialised methods of treatment, and maintain continuity of care for their patients in a way similar to a qualified dental surgeon.

Towards the end of the course, there is increasing emphasis on the interrelationship between the different dental specialities, and on the development of skills in diagnosis and treatment planning. Throughout the whole period of clinical study, students are shown how to apply preventive measures and motivate patients to maintain a high standard of oral health. There is also a two-week period in residence at a district general hospital, and students undertake a six-week elective project that can take them to the far corners of the earth.

Outreach placements provide an opportunity to treat an extended range of patients in community clinics, dental access centres and general dental practices, many of these placements being away from Sheffield.

PS